T0366840

Mental Health Services
for Deaf People

Mental Health Services for Deaf People

Treatment Advances, Opportunities, and Challenges

Benito Estrada Aranda and Ines Sleeboom-van Raaij, *Editors*

Gallaudet University Press
Washington, DC

Gallaudet University Press
Washington, DC 20002
http://gupress.gallaudet.edu

Library of Congress Cataloging-in-Publication Data

World Congress on Mental Health and Deafness (5th : 2012 : Monterrey, Mexico),
author.
  Mental health services for deaf people : treatment advances, opportunities, and
challenges / Benito
Estrada Aranda and Ines Sleeboom-van Raaij, editors.
      p. ; cm.
"This volume presents thirteen papers selected from the presentations at the fifth
World Congress"—
Introduction.
  Includes bibliographical references and index.
ISBN 978-1-56368-654-2 (hardcover : alk. paper) — ISBN 978-1-56368-655-9
(ebook)
I. Estrada Aranda, Benito Daniel, editor. II. Raaij, Ines Sleeboom-van, editor. III.
Title.
  [DNLM: 1. Community Mental Health Services—Congresses. 2. Persons With
Hearing Impairments—
Congresses. 3. Deafness—psychology—Congresses. 4. Mental Disorders—
therapy—Congresses. 5.
Mentally Ill Persons—psychology—Congresses. WA 305.1]
  RC451.4.D4
  362.4'2—dc23
                                                                    201529167

∞ This paper meets the requirements of ANSI/NISO Z39.48-1992 (Permanence of
Paper).

Contents

Acknowledgments

We, the editors of this book, wish to express our appreciation to all of the authors herein for the chapters they contributed. The information they present will be valuable to many professionals in our field.

We especially thank the Mexican Deaf[1] community, as well as the Office of Special Education of the state of Nuevo León, Mexico, and its director, Manuel Antonio García Treviño. We also want to express our appreciation to the Convention and Visitors Office of the state of Nuevo León, Mexico, for its support, advice, and sponsorship of the Fifth World Congress on Mental Health and Deafness. We are especially grateful to Karen A. Tinsley for reviewing the final draft of the book. In addition, we thank both the University Autónoma de Nuevo León and its Department of Psychology for hosting the congress, as well as the staff members who organized the conference. We wish to convey our gratitude to the conference funders and to the dean of the Department of Psychology, Armando Peña Moreno. The work of many people made this book possible; it represents a great effort carried out in a country with no public mental health services for Deaf people and only a few specialized mental health professionals in this field.

Our heartfelt thanks go out to all of you as together we strive to improve the well-being of the Deaf community in Mexico and Deaf communities around the world.

---

1. In this book we refer to Deaf people with a capital *D* to signify those who were born profoundly deaf or lost their hearing before their fourth year of life. These individuals use sign language to communicate and identify themselves as members of the Deaf community.

Introduction: Purpose, Structure, and Contents of the Book

Benito Estrada Aranda
Javier García Muñoz
Ines Sleeboom-van Raaij

Seventeen years have passed since the first World Congress on Mental Health and Deafness at Gallaudet University in Washington, DC, in October 1998. That conference was presided over by Dr. Barbara Brauer and organized in collaboration with the European Society for Mental Health and Deafness. During the intervening years, five more world congresses have been held—in Copenhagen, Denmark (2000); Worcester, South Africa (2005); Brisbane, Australia (2009); Monterrey, Mexico (2012); and, most recently, in Belfast, Ireland (2014). This volume presents thirteen papers selected from the presentations at the fifth World Congress, which was organized by the Department of Psychology at the Autonomous University of Nuevo León (Mexico) and was presided over by Benito Estrada Aranda and Ines Sleeboom-van Raaij. The contributors offer insights and perspectives from eight different countries.

The resulting book is divided into three parts—mental health issues and treatment, deaf populations, and deaf children and their families. In the first part, the contributors take an in-depth look at specific challenges and treatment modalities. Exploring mental health issues and deafness from a human rights perspective, Ana María García García and Javier Muñoz Bravo argue that adequate mental health care should be recognized as a human right and protected by international rules. Ines Sleeboom-van Raaij describes the psychopharmacological treatment of deaf and hard of hearing patients and warns of the frequent and special side effects they experience. Benito Estrada Aranda writes of the challenges and opportunities surrounding the development of mental health and deafness services in countries (e.g., Mexico) that provide no specific public mental health services for deaf people. Lieke Doornkate presents a newly developed treatment in the field of mental health and deafness for families with deaf members: eye movement desensitization and reprocessing (EMDR) therapy. Her chapter is one of the first accounts of this new treatment. Karen Tinsley reviews another new therapeutic approach for use with deaf patients that promises to be a viable and effective option: equine-assisted counseling. The first part closes with a chapter by Irene Leigh on the psychosocial implications of cochlear implants.

Part 2 focuses on deaf populations. In the first chapter, Katerina Antonopoulou, Kika Hadjikakou, and Maria Charalambous examine the relationship between self-esteem and cultural identity among deaf and hard of hearing adults in Greece and Cyprus. Johannes Fellinger addresses the creation, objectives, and services of a clinic in Austria that has been providing public health care to deaf people since 1991. This part concludes with the results of a qualitative study by Poorna Kushalnagar, Melissa Draganac-Hawk, and Donald L. Patrick. These researchers conducted interviews with young deaf and hard of hearing people from Spanish-speaking homes in the United States in an effort to discover the relationship between language differences at home, at school, and in the community, as well as the perceived quality of life for this population.

The third and final part of the book contains four chapters. It begins with Tiejo van Gent's overview of the epidemiology, etiology, and cultural, linguistic, and developmental aspects of mental health and related issues found among deaf children and adolescents. Van Gent follows this up with a discussion of the research on specific psychopathological aspects of mental health symptoms. Joanna Kobosko reports on a study of deaf adolescents with hearing parents, paying special attention to the relationship between a hearing mother and her deaf child and to language development disorders. The volume concludes with a case study of a severely deaf prelocutive child diagnosed as autistic. The authors, Benito Estrada Aranda, Georgina Mitre Fajardo, and Ricardo Canal Bedia, discuss the challenges in these cases, where the symptoms of one condition may mask the symptoms of another.

Taken all together, these chapters explore issues that are important in the specialized area of mental health and deafness. The contributors bring many years of collective experience to the field, and most of them are pioneers of mental health and deafness services in their respective countries as well as members of the European Society for Mental Health and Deafness. They have participated as presenters at the past six world congresses on mental health and deafness.

Mental Health Services for Deaf People

Part 1

Mental Health Issues and Treatment

1

Mental Health Care for Deaf People: An Approach Based on Human Rights

Ana María García García
Javier Muñoz Bravo

Since Deaf people who have a mental illness are often viewed as a minority within a minority, this topic would seem to be of interest to very few people. In fact, the number of professionals interested and/or active in this field is quite small worldwide. However, we believe that the experiences of Deaf people who suffer mistreatment and/or discrimination at the hands of health-care services are universal and therefore not minor. Given that health care is considered a fundamental human right, denial or ignorance of the specific mental health–care needs of Deaf people may be a violation of this right and thus should be of concern to the treating professionals, the governing representative, and every citizen as well.

HEALTH AND HUMAN RIGHTS

In 1946 the right to health was spelled out in the Constitution of the World Health Organization (WHO) as follows: "The enjoyment of the highest attainable health is one of the fundamental rights of every human being without distinction of race, religion, political beliefs, economic or social condition." The right to health care was reaffirmed by the Declaration of Alma-Ata in 1978, by the World Health Declaration, which was adopted by the World Health Assembly in 1998, and by a number of other international and regional human rights instruments.[1]

Because health is a variable beyond the direct control of governing states and depends on a variety of environmental, genetic, cultural, and individual factors, the right to health is not the right to good health or freedom from disease.

The right to health refers to the obligation of states to create conditions that permit all citizens to live as healthily as possible. These include, of course, the guaranteed availability of equitable and appropriate health services, as well as of the primary health-determining conditions, such as access to potable water; adequate sanitation services; a nutritious food supply; appropriate housing; a healthy work environment; and access to education and to information on health issues, including sexual and reproductive health. Established as a fundamental and universal human right that is guaranteed under and protected by international law, the right to health is therefore very important inasmuch as human rights protect individuals and groups of people from actions that undermine their fundamental freedoms and human dignity.

The right to health imposes three types of obligations on the states that ratify them:

- *Respect:* the enjoyment of the right to health
- *Protection* from actions of third parties (with the possible exception of the state) that would interfere with the enjoyment of the right to health
- *Compliance:* the implementation of positive measures to make the right to health a reality by establishing policies and action plans that provide access to health care for all people as soon as possible. States must adopt measures in accordance with the principle of progressive realization. This means that they must go forward as quickly and efficiently as possible, by their own means as well as with international help and cooperation up to the maximum extent of the available resources.

Human rights are interdependent and interconnected. The Vienna Declaration and Programme of Action states the following:[2] "The international community must treat human rights globally in a fair and equal manner, on the same footing, and with the same emphasis . . . [I]t is the duty of States, regardless of their political, economic and cultural systems, to promote and protect all human rights and fundamental freedoms." Since health as a right is affected by other rights having to do with the maintenance of an adequate standard of living, such as access to education or employment, then people who live in poverty or are inadequately educated are more likely to have poorer health than those who enjoy economic security and decent living conditions. It is significant that poverty, inadequate access to education, and other factors that have a negative impact on human rights appear disproportionately among people with disabilities, including Deaf people.

The universality of human rights means they are applicable to everyone worldwide, including people with disabilities and/or mental health problems. Despite the fact that the United Nations resolutions that protect individuals with mental health problems explicitly forbid discrimination against them,[3] these individuals continue to be widely stigmatized and thus are especially susceptible to violation of their human rights as a result of discrimination and increased barriers to medical treatment, housing, education, employment, and so on.

The Human Rights Committee (General Comment[4] no. 14, 2000[5]) sets out the following four evaluation criteria to assess the respect of the right to health:

1. *Availability.* Functioning public health and health-care facilities, goods and services, as well as programmes, have to be available in sufficient quantity . . .
2. *Accessibility.* Health facilities, goods and services have to be accessible to everyone without discrimination, within jurisdiction of the state party. Accessibility has four overlapping dimensions.
   - Non-discrimination: health facilities, goods and services must be accessible to all, especially the most vulnerable or marginalized sections of the population, in law and in fact, without discrimination on any of the prohibited grounds.
   - Physical accessibility: health facilities, goods and services must be within safe physical reach for all sections of the population, especially vulnerable or marginalized groups, such as ethnic minorities and indigenous populations, women, children, adolescents, older persons, persons with disabilities and persons with HIV/AIDS, including in rural areas.
   - Economic accessibility (affordability): health facilities, goods and services must be affordable for all. Payment for health-care services, as well as services related to the underlying determinants of health, has to be based on the principle of equity, ensuring that these services, whether privately or publicly provided, are affordable for all.
   - Information accessibility: accessibility includes the right to seek, receive and impart information and ideas concerning health issues. However, accessibility of information should not impair the right to have personal health data treated with confidentiality.
3. *Acceptability.* All health facilities, goods and services must be respectful of medical ethics and culturally appropriate . . . [and] sensitive to gender and life-cycle requirements, as well as being designed to respect confidentiality and improve the health status of those concerned.
4. *Quality.* . . . Health facilities, goods and services must also be scientifically and medically appropriate and of good quality. This requires, *inter alia,* skilled medical personnel. . . .

In summary, the right to health is a central human right protected by international rules that obligate countries to adopt and implement a national public health strategy. As a universal right and thus applicable to everyone, health should be promoted by national policies that include a participatory and transparent process of review and evaluation and pay particular attention to vulnerable or marginalized groups.

Human Rights, Disability, and Health

In 2001 the United Nations began developing a comprehensive and integral international convention that would protect and promote the rights and the dignity of persons with disabilities.[6] Beginning formally with the Mexican government's appeal to the international community, first at the World Conference against Racism, Racial Discrimination, Xenophobia, and Related Intolerance[7] and later during the fifty-sixth session of the United Nations General Assembly in November 2001, the process of crafting an international treaty aimed at improving the quality of life of persons with disabilities was set in motion.

Thus, the General Assembly of the United Nations decided to establish a special committee[8] with the mission of preparing the International Convention on the Rights of Persons with Disabilities.[9] The text of the convention was adopted by the United Nations General Assembly on December 13, 2006, and opened for signature on March 30, 2007.

The goal of this convention was to ensure that people with disabilities and people without disabilities had equal rights and access to health. In addition to reviewing the existing rights, as discussed earlier, proposals were presented for measures that can be taken by states and civil societies to ensure the reduction or elimination of discrimination against people with disabilities.

Article 25 of the convention refers specifically to health rights. In other words, states are expected to take all appropriate measures to ensure equal access to health services and health-related rehabilitation for persons with disabilities. These proposed measures include the following:

1. Provide persons with disabilities with the same range, quality and standard of free or affordable health care and programmes as provided to other persons . . . ;
2. Provide those health services needed by persons with disabilities specifically because of their disabilities, including early identification and intervention as appropriate, and services designed to minimize and prevent further disabilities, including among children and older persons;
3. Provide these health services as close as possible to people's own communities, including in rural areas;
4. Require health professionals to provide care of the same quality to persons with disabilities as to others, including on the basis of free and informed consent . . . ;
5. Prohibit discrimination against persons with disabilities in the provision of health insurance, and life insurance when such is permitted by national law . . . ;
6. Prevent discriminatory denial of health care or services or food and fluids on the basis of disability.

In summary, the International Convention on the Rights of Persons with Disabilities can be considered an official document whose purpose is to ensure the full enactment of human rights for persons with disabilities.

DEAF PEOPLE AND MENTAL HEALTH SERVICES

The foregoing discussion also applies to the health-care provisions for Deaf people; in this section we provide further comment on the mental health issues for this population. All too often, Deaf people experience two main types of discrimination: direct and indirect.

Direct Discrimination

Direct discrimination is the different or less favorable treatment experienced by a person with a disability in comparison to the treatment received by a person without a disability in the same or a similar context. The following are illustrations:

1. *Access to information.* The most fundamental area in which Deaf people experience discrimination is communication, the lack of which denies them access to needed information, especially during medical diagnosis, treatment, and aftercare. Although diagnosis may be enhanced by diagnostic tests, biopsies, X-rays, endoscopy, ECGs, palpation, auscultation, and so on, it is still essential to interview patients directly, make note of their perceptions, mood, and behavior, and communicate with others who know them. This is especially important in mental health situations, and it is essential to communicate with patients directly by using a shared communication system.
2. *Communication constraints.* Since most health professionals are unfamiliar with sign language and may even refuse to accept the use of sign language, interpreters, and other assistive resources, the risk of misdiagnosis and treatment errors increases.

    Good mental health care for Deaf persons tends to require at least twice as much time and twice as many personnel as required for hearing people.[10] Even when Deaf individuals are treated for about the same length of time as hearing people, they may still receive lower-quality care. Furthermore, with rare exception (e.g., Wechsler Intelligence Scale for Children, 4th ed.; Rhode Island Test of Language Structure), psychodiagnostic tests (e.g., IQ, personality) are designed for and standardized on the general hearing population; thus, without proper adaptation or accommodation, the use of these instruments with Deaf patients may increase the chance of errors in diagnosis.
3. *Confidentiality.* Since health professionals are often more likely to provide medical or mental health information to relatives or other significant people in a Deaf person's life—even without the patient's consent—there is a higher risk of violation of confidentiality.
4. *Disinformation.* Deaf patients often do not receive adequate information about their condition (diagnosis, prognosis, or proper care). Examples of disinformation, with potentially serious consequences for the (right to) health of Deaf patients, include the following:

- Inappropriate medication or treatment management due to insufficient information about dosage or possible side effects
- Deaf patients' receipt of inadequate information at discharge about appropriate aftercare, which puts them at high risk of reentry. This is compounded by the fact that many Deaf patients have no opportunity to access social or similar resources to obtain this information if it is not provided during treatment.
- Most informed-consent forms signed by Deaf persons before any medical intervention occurs may not be valid because the information on the forms is presented in an incomprehensible format, leaving these individuals in a situation of helplessness with regard to medical decisions.

5. *Physical accessibility.* Health facilities often provide insufficient accommodations to the needs of Deaf patients, particularly with respect to visual accessibility (e.g., they may use loudspeakers or alarms without visual indicators or text). Many health-care facilities are geographically too far away from Deaf patients and their interpreters. Lack of available interpreting services, along with the scarcity of additional specialized resources for Deaf people, can also affect the health issues of these patients.

6. *Isolation.* Even though admission to a psychiatric unit is difficult for anyone, it can be especially so for Deaf patients since, in many cases, they are the only ones admitted to a given unit. Because of the additional difficulties of finding Deaf or hearing professionals who know sign language, the result may be the de facto isolation of these patients and the increased risk of patient abuse due to the patients' inadequate understanding of institutional protocol and their greater vulnerability. Moreover, Deaf patients usually receive few visits from Deaf friends or relatives due to the barriers the latter encounter.

7. *Health professionals' training issues.* Historically, health professionals have been trained to view disability from a medical perspective.[11] In other words, they are instructed to understand deafness as a disease that needs to be eliminated. Common prejudices held by many health professionals include the belief that Deaf people are distrustful, less intelligent, and/or more unhappy than hearing people. The discomfort that health professionals experience when working with Deaf people or dealing with the related communication issues may lead to earlier discharges from their services or premature referrals to other professionals.

Indirect Discrimination

Indirect discrimination is the occurrence—as the result of a seemingly neutral act or disposition—of a disproportionate disadvantage or negative effect for persons with a disability relative to persons who have no disability. For example, certain policies may inadvertently bring about more adverse effects for a disadvantaged group, such as Deaf people, than for a nondisadvantaged group. Very basic, every-day examples of indirect discrimination may include the following:

- Rigidity of the health services bureaucracy. Every process—from appointment requests to payment for medical services—is designed for hearing people. Deaf people often must use complex phone systems to make an appointment, fill out complicated written forms, deal with insurance or public employees who do not use sign language or an alternate communication system, and so on. Even though the bureaucracy is intended to ensure that the system provides equal access to health care for all, it may fail to do so for Deaf people.
- Inadequate visual information. In many cases the obligation to provide architectural uniformity throughout a hospital or other health facility actually makes it more difficult for Deaf people to navigate offices and hallways. Using distinctive signs and colors to identify the location of various services (e.g., specialized services for Deaf people) would be more helpful and improve equality of access.
- Although the law in many countries attempts to guarantee quality health services for all citizens, this requirement may in fact backfire against minorities such as Deaf people by focusing only on the *context* of providing equal services while neglecting the *content;* that is, the general practice or application may not result in equal benefits. Rationales against providing adaptations or accommodations (e.g., specialized or increased staff; a variety of systems of communication access) include the argument that doing so would violate the law and create a different kind of discrimination against other citizens.
- Indirect discrimination may also be evident in the recruitment of Deaf professionals for either general or specialized mental health–care units. Deaf professionals are expected to meet the same requirements as hearing professionals, including passing the same entrance exams and obtaining the same degrees, often without appropriate accommodations.

To sum up, health laws that are designed to protect the health of the general population and guarantee access to health services may exclude, discriminate against, or treat patients and professionals with disabilities less favorably by failing to provide appropriate accessibility and accommodation.

OVERCOMING DISCRIMINATION: TOWARD A GOOD MODEL OF MENTAL HEALTH CARE FOR DEAF PEOPLE

What result can the application of the United Nations Convention on the Rights of Persons with Disabilities have for Deaf people in the domain of mental health? How can we eliminate the discrimination that Deaf patients currently suffer? And what steps should we take in order to implement mental health services that adequately meet the needs of Deaf people in those countries where such services do not yet exist? How can we defend the already existing services?

To achieve equality in the domain of mental health for Deaf people necessarily involves treating them in a different way. It is essential to introduce measures of positive discrimination, such as specific mental health services, and differentiating policies to reduce the existing disparity between the treatment that health services provide to hearing people and to Deaf people.

It is very important to emphasize that positive discrimination measures do not differentiate between the general population and groups of people with disabilities for two reasons: First, any measure of differentiation that privileges certain people does not entail the negative features of underestimation, contempt, and even less the stigmatization of those who are excluded, something that unfair traditional discriminations did entail. Moreover, there is evidence that improvement in medical care for people with disabilities has a positive impact on other minorities and the population in general. Second, the goal of the positive discrimination measures is the overcoming of serious inequalities in the past, with the result that those measures achieve fairer relations among different groups of people.

We now list some general measures that should be included in a comprehensive mental health plan for Deaf people in those countries interested in improving the situation of Deaf people with mental health problems. Such a plan must provide a global response to the needs of this group in the domain of mental health with regard to equality of opportunities and accessibility. Furthermore, this plan must be developed with the active participation of organizations representing Deaf people. Special attention should be paid to Deaf women with mental health problems since they might be subject to multiple forms of discrimination on the grounds of gender, disability, and illness.

Our recommended measures are the following:

1. Analyze in detail the status of health care for Deaf people in rural areas. Design and implement a specific program that has sufficient resources to achieve equality of opportunity regardless of where these people live.
2. Design and implement a comprehensive policy of both universal accessibility and elimination of architectural, attitudinal, and communication barriers that Deaf people encounter in health care. This policy must promote the development of effective, concrete actions.
3. Eliminate administrative and bureaucratic red tape and provide helping mechanisms for Deaf people (technical support, specialized professional support, etc.).
4. Guarantee access to complete medical information through the use of a comprehensible language and/or other format for Deaf people as well as by eliminating all barriers in health facilities and procedures. Promote sign language instruction for medical and administrative staff in order to promote universal accessibility in communication. Patients must have access to all information

concerning their rights as patients and users of the health-care system, their medical history and documents, and procedures for giving informed consent.

5. Promote and protect interpreters of sign language and guarantee Deaf people's access to interpreters who are adequately trained to work in the domain of mental health.

6. Encourage health and social services professionals' initial and continuing education on psychopathological disorders in order to prevent or detect such problems early on and treat them accordingly.

7. Raise awareness in and encourage the training of health professionals regarding persons with disabilities and specifically on the idiosyncrasies and particularities of the Deaf community in order to eliminate prejudices and stereotypes.

8. In emergencies services, design and implement a universally accessible system that enables all Deaf persons to communicate (by email, short message service [SMS], sign language interpreters, etc.).

9. Encourage the integration of Deaf people as professional health-care employees. In this sense, the basic criteria and conditions of entrance exams must be established in order to make it possible for potential Deaf professionals to pass them. The same must be extended to specialized medical training.

10. Promote awareness campaigns for the general population by means of education efforts aimed at eliminating prejudices, stereotypes, and other attitudes that undermine the right of people to be equal, thus promoting respect for and coexistence with Deaf people and people with mental disorders.

11. Encourage research on Deaf people's mental health in its epidemiological and clinical aspects.

12. As a quality criterion of the health-care system, focus on diversity awareness specifically with regard to people with disabilities.

CONCLUSIONS

The right to health is a human right that is recognized and protected by international rules. Nations are obliged to respect, protect, and take measures to guarantee this right to their citizens, including Deaf persons. They must ensure the availability of health services that are accessible (i.e., nondiscriminatory, as well as geographically, physically, economically, and informatively obtainable), ethical, respectful of cultures, and of good quality.

In 2006 the General Assembly of the United Nations approved the International Convention on the Rights of the Persons with Disabilities. Its purpose is to protect and ensure the full and equal enjoyment of human rights and fundamental freedoms by all persons with disabilities. Article 25 of the convention refers specifically to health. Nations recognize that persons with disabilities have the right to enjoy the highest attainable standard of health without discrimination.

Most Deaf people, and especially those with mental disorders, suffer both direct and indirect discrimination when they seek health care. It is essential to support the implementation of positive discrimination measures in order to ensure that Deaf people receive the correct care in the domain of mental health. The approach according to which health is a human right must become the main argument in supporting the implementation of new mental health services for Deaf people and in defending the existing ones.

The first step to take in achieving good-quality mental health services for Deaf people is to demand the proper enforcement of the law within the applicable legal framework for human rights. We must therefore promote effective equal opportunities for people with disabilities and the elimination of discriminatory situations in accordance with the UN Convention on the Rights of Persons with Disabilities. We must demand its enforcement in those countries that have ratified it and advocate for its ratification or signature by those countries that have not yet done so.

Notwithstanding the existence of these international instruments, the main obstacle to the protection of the human rights of people with disabilities is the fact that most countries do not yet recognize the discrimination that their own citizens are subjected to. To some extent, this difficulty has been overcome by international organizations such as the European Commission of Human Rights, the Inter-American Commission on Human Rights, and the International Criminal Court, not to mention the work of NGOs worldwide, which promote the protection of human rights and the elimination of all forms of discrimination.

Therefore, in order to overcome the bias experienced by Deaf people with mental disorders it is essential that Deaf people—associations, families, and professionals—insist that as many countries as possible ratify the convention and demand its effective enforcement. It is also necessary that both the legal framework and public health policies pay closer and more sustained attention to issues such as health and deafness, especially in the domain of mental health. Moreover, it is vital to implement specific mental health services for Deaf people. These must be accessible and involve professionals—both Deaf and hearing—who are well trained in both clinical and communicative aspects of dealing with Deaf patients. Proper health care for Deaf people with mental disorders is an ethical issue, not a matter of cost effectiveness. It is the responsibility of those who are familiar with the status quo to insist that the existing inequalities be corrected.

NOTES

1. The right to health is recognized as a human right in numerous international instruments. For instance, paragraph 1 of Article 25 of the Universal Declaration of Human Rights (1948) states that "Everyone has the right to a standard of living adequate for the health and well-being of himself and of his family, including food, clothing, housing and medical care and necessary social services." In addition, the International Covenant on Economic, Social,

and Cultural Rights (1966) contains the most complete article on the right to health in international legislation on human rights. There, paragraph 1 of Article 12 explains that states recognize "the right of everyone to enjoy the highest possible standard of physical and mental health," and paragraph 2 of the same article lists a few measures as examples. These measures "will be adopted by the States Parties . . . in order to ensure the total effectiveness of this right."

Moreover, the right to health is recognized in other instruments, such as the International Convention on the Elimination of All Forms of Racial Discrimination (1963), the Convention on the Elimination of All Forms of Discrimination against Women (1979), and the Convention on the Rights of the Child (1989), as well as a few regional instruments of human rights, such as the European Social Charter (1961) in its revised form, the 1981 African Charter on Human and Peoples' Rights, and the Additional Protocol of the American Convention on Human Rights: Economic, Social, and Cultural Rights (1988), which has been in force since 1999. Likewise, the right to health was proclaimed by the Commission on Human Rights and further treated in the 1993 Vienna Declaration and Programme of Action and other international instruments.

2. Vienna Declaration and Programme of Action, approved by the World Conference on Human Rights, Vienna, June 14–25, 1993, paragraph 5 (A/CONF.137/23 of the United Nations General Assembly).

3. Principle 1 of the United Nations General Assembly resolution 46/119, February 18, 1992, on the protection of persons with mental illness and the improvement of mental health care.

4. The Human Rights Committee publishes its interpretation of the content of human rights provisions in the form of general comments on thematic issues.

5. Substantive issues arising in the implementation of the international covenant on economic, social, and cultural rights (General Comment no. 14, 2000). The right to the highest attainable standard of health (article 12 of the International Covenant on Economic, Social, and Cultural Rights).

6. In this process several actors took part: state members, UN agencies, the UN special rapporteur on disability, national human rights institutions, and nongovernmental organizations (NGOs), among which organizations of persons with disabilities and their families played a leading role.

7. Durban, South Africa, August 31–September 8, 2001.

8. Resolution 56/168, December 19, 2001.

9. www.un.org/disabilities/documents/convention/convoptprot-e.pdf.

10. Ines Sleeboom-van Raaij, *The Importance of a Specialized Mental Health Service for the Deaf*, paper presented at the Fifth World Congress on Mental Health and Deafness, Monterrey, Mexico, 2012.

11. Traditionally, disability has been understood as the expression of a deficiency simply from a functional point of view and/or a person's activity. That is to say, disability was defined as a limitation derived from the endurance of a physical, mental, intellectual, and/or sensorial deficit. The medical model applied to disability is obviously centered on the malfunction of a specific mechanism (physical, sensorial, and/or intellectual) and presents an obvious idea: Disability is a medical condition that requires some kind of remedy.

BIBLIOGRAPHY

Baker, K. L., & Baker, F. (2011). Assessing intellectual disability with Deaf people. *International Journal of Deafness and Mental Health, 1*(1), 22–35.

Closing the gap in a generation: Health equity through action on the social determinants of health. (2008). Geneva: World Health Organization.

Constitution of the World Health Organization. (1948). Geneva: World Health Organization. Retrieved April 9, 2015, from http://apps.who.int/gb/bd/PDF/bd47/EN/constitution-en.pdf

Declaration of Alma-Ata. World Health Organization. (1978). Retrieved April 9, 2015, from http://www.euro.who.int/__data/assets/pdf_file/0009/113877/E93944.pdf

Drum, C. E., Krahn, G. L., Peterson, J. J., Horner-Johnson, W., & Newton, K. (2009). Health of people with disabilities: Determinants and disparities. In C. E. Drum, G. Krahn, & H. Bersani (Eds.), *Disability and public health* (pp. 125–144). Washington, DC: American Public Health Association.

Editorial: The health of deaf people: Communication breakdown. (2012, March 17). *Lancet, 379,* 977.

Fellinger, J., Holzinger, D., & Pollard, R. (2012, March 17). Mental health of deaf people. *Lancet, 379,* 1037–1044.

Huber, M., Stanciole, A., Wahlbeck, K., Tamsma, N., Torres, F., Jelfs, E., & Bremner, J. (2008). *Quality in and equality of access to healthcare services.* Brussels: European Commission.

Lagarde, M., Haines, A., & Palmer, N. (2009). The impact of conditional cash transfers on health outcomes and use of health services in low- and middle-income countries. *Cochrane Database of Systematic Reviews (Online),* 4CD008137- PMID:19821444.

Lord, J. E., Guernsey, K. N., Balfe, J. M., Karr, V. L., & Flowers, N. (Eds.). (2007). *Human rights. YES! Action and advocacy on the rights of persons with disabilities.* Minneapolis: University of Minnesota, Human Rights Resource Center.

Mental health and development: Targeting people with mental health conditions as a vulnerable group. (2010). Geneva: World Health Organization.

Mental health systems in selected low- and middle-income countries: A WHO-AIMS cross-national analysis. (2009). Geneva: World Health Organization.

Ohre, B., von Tetzchner, S., & Falkum, E. (2011). Deaf adults and mental health: A review of recent research on the prevalence and distribution of psychiatric symptoms and disorders in the prelingually Deaf adult population. *International Journal of Deafness and Mental Health, 1*(1), 3–22.

Prince, M., Patel, V., Saxena, S., Maj, M., Maselko, J., Phillips, M. R., & Rahman, A. (2007). No health without mental health. *Lancet, 370,* 859–877. doi:10.1016/S0140-6736(07)61238-0 PMID:17804063.

Tomlinson, M., Swartz, L., Officer, A., Chan, K. Y., Rudan, I., & Shekhar, S. (2009). Research priorities for health of people with disabilities: An expert opinion exercise. *Lancet, 374,* 1857–1862. doi:10.1016/S0140-6736(09)61910-3 PMID:19944866.

United Nations Convention on the Rights of Persons with Disabilities. (2006). Geneva: United Nations. Retrieved April 9, 2015, from http://www.un.org/disabilities/convention/conventionfull.shtml

World Health Assembly Resolution WHA51.12: Health promotion. (1998, May 16). Retrieved April 9, 2015, from http://www.who.int/healthpromotion/wha51-12/en/

World Health Report 2010. (2010). *Health systems financing: The path to universal coverage.* Geneva: World Health Organization.Ana María García García and Javier Muñoz Bravo

2

Important Issues in the Psychopharmacological Treatment of Deaf and Hard of Hearing People with Mental Health Disorders: Theory and Practice

Ines Sleeboom-van Raaij

Deaf and hard of hearing people are not a group of patients with a specific mental or physical disorder but rather a heterogeneous group of people within society for whom one sense organ is not working properly.

In many countries around the world diagnosis and treatment of deaf and hard of hearing people with mental health problems in a specialized facility is still an unfulfilled wish. In the past 50 years services and networks have been developed by pioneers in several countries in Europe, North and South America, South Africa, Australia, and Japan (Queensland Health, 2008; du Feu & Fergusson, 2003; Denmark, 1994; Sleeboom-van Raaij, 1991, 1999; Basilier, 1973; Remvig, 1969; Rainer & Altshuler, 1966).

During that time, however, no specific psychopharmacological research was carried out on deaf and hard of hearing patients (Munro, Knox, & Lowe, 2008; Sleeboom-van Raaij, 1997). The experience of other colleagues in the field has often been the only guideline. In international meetings specific and severe side effects of psychiatric medication have been cited (Sleeboom-van Raaij, 1997). The cause of these specific side effects is still unknown, as they occur in the whole group of deaf people, although it can be assumed that they are more prevalent among specific causes of deafness, such as brain damage and infectious diseases. Factors that contribute to particular mental health disorders related to prenatal rubella deafness (Brown et al., 2001, 2005; Chess, Korn, & Fernandez, 1971) and deafness due to other prenatal infections (Brown et al., 2005; Buka, 2001) and the consequences for the psychopharmacological treatment are still unknown.

Often hearing mental health providers assume that a "hearing" service and hearing professionals working together with a sign language interpreter for deaf patients should be sufficient (Landsberger & Diaz, 2010; du Feu & Fergusson, 2003; Ebert & Heckerling, 1995). However, both psychopharmacological treatment and psychoeducation of deaf people require specialized knowledge of many aspects related to deafness that can influence this part of the psychiatric treatment (Fellinger, Holzinger, & Pollard, 2012; Black & Glickman, 2006; Gorlin, Toriello, & Cohen, 1995). To understand these factors and interpret the questions and answers adequately specialized professionals are needed (Landsberger & Diaz, 2010; du Feu & Fergusson, 2003).

GENERAL ASPECTS OF PSYCHOPHARMACOLOGY IN MENTAL HEALTH AND DEAFNESS

In adult psychiatry the results of what went physically, psychologically, socially, mentally, and educationally wrong in the life of the patient are evident. Frequently observed biopsychosocial factors can show the hazards, the risks, and the positive effects of these factors on the mental health of the individual (van Gent, 2012; Hindley & Kitson, 2000).

Experience has taught that several aspects that are directly or indirectly related to deafness play a role in the diagnostic process and treatment of deaf and hard of hearing patients (van Gent, 2012; Fellinger et al., 2012; Sleeboom-van Raaij & Knoppert-van der Klein 2003; du Feu & Fergusson, 2003). During psychopharmacological treatment the following factors are important: aetiology (cause) of the deafness, age of onset, additional handicaps and comorbidity, means and level of communication and language abilities, general knowledge, and cultural issues. For a summary, see Table 1.

Language Abilities

Unfortunately, not all deaf people are able to learn to sign, lip-read, or read adequately (Landsberger & Diaz, 2010). Black and Glickman (2006), experienced clinicians in the field of mental health and deafness, found that two-thirds of their deaf inpatients were dysfluent in any language. Several of the deaf inpatients in the Netherlands have severely limited communication skills such as some signing, gesturing, and/or inadequate lipreading and speech; some of the patients had no language skills at all. These limited language skills were caused by the following:

- delayed diagnosis of the deafness (doctor's delay, parents' delay)
- nonacceptance/denial of the deafness by the parents and other family members

TABLE 1.   Essential Information (in Addition to the Psychiatric Diagnosis) for
            the Medical Professional prior to Prescribing Psychopharmacological
            Medication to Deaf and Hard of Hearing Patients

Aetiology of the deafness
Kind of deafness
Age of onset
Additional handicaps
Co-morbidity

Communication level and mode of the patient
Language abilities of the patient
General knowledge level of the patient
Psychosocial aspects of deafness

Psychiatric history
Addiction (Substance abuse)
Psychopharmacological medication (current)
Psychopharmacological history
Side effects history

Family history:
*psychiatric
*somatic
*pharmacological
Country of origin

Somatic history
Somatic medication (current)
Somatic pharmacological history
Other current medical treatment
Allergic reactions

Physical examination
RR, pulse, temperature, weight, length, waistlength
Laboratory tests
Contact with general practitioner or other medical specialist to obtain information

---

- nonacceptance of the deafness in the community
- noncommunicative family or other environment in which the individual grew up
- mainstreaming of the individual in a hearing school without special provisions
- lack of schooling

In the Netherlands, patients specifically of foreign origin, such as those from
the Middle East, Africa, Surinam, and the Dutch Caribbean, are highly represented in this group. Their limited development of language and communication and/or a noncommunicative environment can also hinder the acquisition of
general knowledge through incidental learning. In these circumstances, communication with the patient during the assessment interview and in treatment and

psychoeducation is complex. Difficult terminology and complex sentences should be avoided (Landsberger & Diaz, 2010; Chaveiro, Celeno Porto, & Alves Barbosa, 2009; Lezzoni, O'Day, Killeen, & Harker, 2004; du Feu & Fergusson, 2003). Barriers can be overcome, however, by making use of a deaf relay interpreter. In addition, drawings, photographs, pictures, and taking sufficient time will enhance the communication with these patients.

Ideally, the medical professional treating deaf patients should be able to sign or at least use a sign language interpreter trained specifically in working with deaf mental health patients (Fellinger et al., 2012; Pereira, 2010; Lezzoni et al., 2004; du Feu & Fergusson, 2003; Steinberg, Sullivan, & Loew, 1998; Steinberg, Barnett, Meador, Wiggins, & Zazove, 2006).

Many deaf patients, however, encounter a cultural and linguistic barrier to health and mental health services (Pereira, 2010; Lezzoni et al., 2004; Steinberg et al., 1998, 2002; Steinberg et al., 2006; Zazove et al., 1993). Negative experiences and avoidance or nonuse of the health services were reported (Pereira, 2010; Steinberg et al., 2006; Lezzoni et al., 2004). As a result, they have an evident lack of general health knowledge and little understanding of screening and the purpose of prescribed medication (Pereira, 2010; Lezzoni et al., 2004; Steinberg et al., 2002, 2006). In the Netherlands inpatients often mentioned that they had not visited their general practitioner for a long time due to communication problems and the practitioner's misunderstanding of their complaints. A severely depressed inpatient mentioned in the admission interview that she had had no contact with her general practitioner for several years for this reason. The laboratory tests in the hospital showed a nonfunctional thyroid gland.

Not all patients are aware of their own communication barriers in their contact with medical professionals. The following case histories illustrate this:

∾

Accompanied by his father, a very hard of hearing, independently living, 26-year-old man with hereditary deafness and autism visited his internal medicine specialist. His form of communication was lipreading, speech, and Dutch with signs. He refused to use an interpreter during doctor's visits. For his hereditary disorder he was required to take calcium supplements for quite some time. The specialist discussed with him and his father the possibility of slowly tapering off on the use of the supplement. However, he misread the advice from the specialist and, at home, immediately stopped taking the calcium. Three days later his mental health-care worker visited him and found him sitting in a chair in a pre-comatose state, mentally deteriorated, jittery, and dizzy, with muscle cramps and no proper reaction to questions. He was admitted to the hospital just in time to prevent his death.

∾

A 60-year-old, prelingually deaf inpatient with bipolar disorder had a sudden attack of angioedema, a recurrent, noninflammatory swelling of the skin on the face and hands and of the mucosal tissues of the upper respiratory and gastrointestinal tracts. Laryngeal edema can be life threatening, and the pain of the gastrointestinal attacks may be incapacitating (Lin & Chen, 2010; Kulthanan, Jiamton, Boochangkool, & Jongjarearnprasert, 2007). Although this had happened before at home, the patient's general practitioner had not informed him of the cause or the consequences of his severe attacks of angioedema, how to handle a relapse, or the necessity of informing the patient's other medical professionals of his condition. The communication barrier between physician and patient clearly played an important role.

≈

For the mental health professional who is treating deaf or hard of hearing patients it is essential to be acquainted with these communication and language aspects and to recognize the psychosocial and physical consequences they can have for these individuals.

ETIOLOGY OF DEAFNESS, ADDITIONAL HANDICAPS, AND COMORBIDITY

Often deaf patients do not know the precise cause of their deafness. In the Netherlands schools are obliged by law to destroy all files after pupils have left. Due to this policy, important information is lost. From one of the adult patients with CHARGE syndrome (Jyonouchi, McDonald-McGinn, Bale, Zackai, & Sullivan, 2009), a very complex syndrome, no test results or physical data were available, which complicated treatment immensely. Some of the patients' psychiatric or psychological problems stem from the etiology of the deafness. In prenatal rubella, cytomegalovirus, and toxoplasmosis, a higher frequency of nonaffective psychosis is observed (Brown, Cohen, et al., 2001; Brown, Schaefer, et al., 2005; Brown, 2011, 2012; Buka et al., 2001). Prenatal rubella can cause congenital deafness and blindness, as well as cardiovascular diseases, hypothyroidism, and aggressive behavior in adolescence (Dammeyer, 2010; Banatvala & Brown, 2004).The effect of the prenatal rubella infection in later life is often unknown to the patient and the family, although several physical symptoms may be observed (Duszak 2009; Barnett, 2012; Van Nunen-Schrauwen & Schoenmaker, 2007). For example, in treating a depression with antidepressive medication, a medical practitioner needs to know whether the patient suffers from cardiovascular abnormalities due to hereditary, congenital, or pre- and postnatal infectious illnesses.

Patients with deafness due to infectious diseases such as encephalomen-ingitis or brain damage have a seizurogenic condition and are vulnerable to epileptogenic medication. Seizures triggered by psychotropic drugs are a dose-dependent adverse effect (Pisani, Oteri, Costa, Di Raimondo, & Di Perri, 2002). Clozapine, chlorpromazine, and phenothiazines have a relatively high seizuro-genic potential, while maprotiline, clomipramine, and tricyclic antidepressants have intermediate seizurogenic potential. Other antipsychotic drugs, such as haloperidol, pimozide, risperidone, and several other antidepressants such as bupropion present a relatively low risk (Ruffmann, Bogliun, & Beghi, 2006; Pisani et al., 2002).

Symptoms and signs of somatic diseases are important to diagnose, as physi-cal illness and mortality in general occur more frequently in people with mental health disorders (Korkeila et al., 2013). In the past, untreated major somatic disor-ders such as epilepsy, hyper- or hypothyroidism, vision disturbances, and anemia were often observed in deaf psychiatric inpatients. Physical examination can be of great value in excluding physical causes of the psychiatric symptoms, treating so-matic disorders, and preventing physical problems during psychopharmacologi-cal treatment.

Knowledge of literature regarding applications of psychopharmacological drugs, their effects, side effects, contraindications, and interactions with other medications is for the medical professional a condition sine qua non, especially in the treatment of deaf people (Moleman & Birkenhäger, 2008; van Harten, 2000, 1998; Sleeboom-van Raaij & Knoppert-van der Klein, 2003).

THE EFFECTS AND SIDE EFFECTS OF MEDICATION ON DEAF AND HARD OF HEARING PATIENTS

Specific Side Effects in Mental Health and Deafness

Side effects may be more prevalent in deaf patients than in hearing patients and may also be more frequent, more intense, or are more troublesome. One reason for this may be the same brain damage that initially caused the deafness, but side effects have also been observed in cases of genetic deafness and other disorders. Moreover, often patients are unable to identify the side effects, do not make the connection between the medication and the adverse reactions, or are unable to express the symptoms they experience due to limited language ability.

Specific Side Effects of Antipsychotic Medication

In the group of patients shown in Table 2, none were able to describe the course of their side effects.

TABLE 2. Side Effects of Antipsychotic Medication on Eight Deaf or Hard of Hearing Patients

Patient Gender Age Origin	Cause of deafness	Mental disorder	Medication	Effect of medication	Side effects	Approach 1	Approach 2
1. Female 25 years African-Dutch	Prenatal Rubella	Schizophrenia paranoid type Mental retardation	Zuclopenthixol Trihexiphenidyl	Insufficient, still paranoid and very aggressive	Walked with arms to the ground (gorilla-like) Fell over when cycling	Lowering dosis: psychotic symptoms increased Other antipsychotic medication (a.o.haloperidol): insufficient effect, same side effects	Clozapine: symptoms and side effects disappeared Can ride a bicycle
2. Male 61 years Caucasian	Meningitis	Schizophrenia paranoid type	Zuclopenthixol Trihexiphenidyl	Sufficient	Extremely inactive, no communication, no desire to walk, sedated, no communication possible	Lowering dosis: psychotic symptoms increased	Olanzapine: alert, side effects disappeared Communication much better: demonstrated symptoms of claudicatio intermittens could be treated.

(continued)

TABLE 2. Side Effects of Antipsychotic Medication on Eight Deaf or Hard of Hearing Patients (*continued*)

Patient Gender Age Origin	Cause of deafness	Mental disorder	Medication	Effect of medication	Side effects	Approach 1	Approach 2
3. Male 25 years Caucasian	Rubella deafness	Schizophrenia paranoid type Impulsivity Aggressive disorder Mental retardation	Zuclopenthixol	Sufficient	Unable to walk: wheelchair necessary	Olanzapine Side effects disappeared	
4. Male 61 years Caucasian	Meningitis	Schizophrenia Parkinsonism (untreated at admission)	Zuclopenthixol Depot at admission	Moderate	Cannot walk more than 2 m, Legs collapsed beneath him Inert, limited communication	Olanzapine: walks normally	
5. Male 28 years North African	Hereditary deafness	Autism, Obsessive Compulsive symptoms Mental retardation Walks on tiptoes with spastic feet	Zuclopenthixol	Moderate	Walks almost normally		

(*continued*)

Patient Gender Age Origin	Cause of deafness	Mental disorder	Medication	Effect of medication	Side effects	Approach 1	Approach 2
6. Female 60 years Caucasian	Late deafness CVA with hemiparesis	Psychotic Disorder NOS	Haloperidol	Moderate	Cannot walk since haloperidol	Not yet treated, clinical discussion necessary due to somatic diseases	
7. Male 30 years Caucasian	Meningitis	Schizophrenia Cannabis abuse	Zuclopenthixol depot	Sufficient	After depot medication 2 days extremely sedated, otherwise sleepy during the day, no energy, tired	Oral medication: poor adherence, psychotic symptoms increased	Paliperidon depot + oral side effects disappeared
8. Male 35 years North African	Unknown	Schizophrenia Cannabis abuse	Zuclopenthixol depot (max dosis)	Insufficient-moderate	After depot medication extremely sedated, sleeping long hours, and inert in between	Paliperidon depot: + oral paliperidon: insufficient effect Side effects disappeared	Zuclopenthixol orally added: Alert and sufficient antipsychotic effect

Table 2, which presents eight case histories of both in- and outpatients, illustrates the specific side effects that deaf patients sometimes experience with antipsychotic medication. All of these patients' psychotic disorders or schizophrenia were difficult to treat and required antipsychotic medication to prevent psychotic symptoms and aggressive behavior. Some of them showed extreme muscle weakness and were unable to walk a short distance or even at all. The literature about side effects and antipsychotic medication with motoric side effects describes the extrapyramidal syndrome (EPS), tardive dyskinesia, and the malignant neuroleptic syndrome. The EPS includes dystonias, Parkinsonism, and akathisia. These descriptions, however, fail to mention muscle weakness (Kamin, Manwani, & Hughes, 2000).

Muscle weakness is also not included in the UKU side-effect rating scale, the Glasgow Antipsychotic Side-Effect Scale (GASS), and the Monitoring of Side Effects Scale (MOSES). Only the MOSES mentions weakness in combination with fatigue (Lingjaerde, Ahlfors, Bech, Dencker, & Elgen, 1987; Waddell & Taylor, 2008; Kalachnik, 1988, 1999). In his cross-sectional study, Vancampfort (2013) describes the relationship between impaired health-related muscular fitness and a reduced walking capacity in patients with schizophrenia. He finds that advanced age, extended illness, a higher BMI, and current physical activity level are independent predictors of muscular fitness, and with caution he adds that a metabolic syndrome causes decreased health-influenced muscle fitness. He finds no relationship between health-related muscular fitness and current antipsychotic medication and EPS. The probability of adverse effects of antipsychotic medication, however, has not been examined by its discontinuation (Naranjo et al., 1981).

Vancampfort's (2013) findings on the effects of medication contrast with our findings, in which the second, third, and fourth patient started walking again after their medication was changed. In the first patient, changing the medication to clozapine helped her resume a normal posture and improved her motoric functioning. For the seventh and eighth patients, a change of medication had a significant positive effect on their activity level, sleeping habits, and sports activities. The hypertonic muscles of the fifth patient's feet improved as a side effect of the antipsychotic medication on the tonus of these muscles.

Only through thorough observation and examination was it discovered that the fourth patient's collapse on the floor was not caused by a conversion disorder as the "hearing" unit had diagnosed but by a side effect of the antipsychotic medication. When his medication was changed from zuclopenthixol to olanzapine, he exhibited improvement in walking and mental functioning. Olanzapine was chosen over clozapine because of the observed myotoxicity and neurotoxicity of clozapine in the literature (Reznik et al., 2000).

Although seven of the eight patients used zuclopenthixol, haloperidol can have a similar effect, as was seen in patients 1 and 6.

Specific Side Effect of Antidepressant Medication

Increased perspiration is an unpleasant, persistent side effect of antidepressant medication in 10% of the patients using selective serotonin reuptake inhibitors (SSRIs) and 14% of tricyclic antidepressants (Trindade, Menon, Topfer, & Coloma, 2008). Increased perspiration is prominent in the face (95%) and the scalp (62%) (Mago, Thase, & Rovner, 2013). This side effect is not always recognized by the patient as such (Marcy & Britton, 2005). Perspiration itself is a sympatic reaction induced by the hypothalamus when stimulated by a high environmental or body temperature (Marcy & Britton, 2005). The physiological mechanism of excessive perspiration with antidepressant medication is unclear (ibid.; Butt, 1989). The result of this side effect for deaf and hard of hearing patients is illustrated in Table 3.

For deaf and hard of hearing patients, increased perspiration on the face and scalp is a serious side effect (Sleeboom-van Raaij, 2010). Excessive sweating can cause damage to the hearing aid or cochlear implant by a short-circuit or oxidation, or the perspiration fluid can make it impossible to wear the hearing aid or implant. The sound produced by the hearing aid may become distorted or even inaudible. For one patient the hyperhidrosis meant social isolation as he was afraid to show his extreme sweating during communication with others.

Increased perspiration can be treated by reducing the dosage, discontinuing the medication, or changing the antidepressant (Mago et al., 2013, 2007; Shinohara, 2009; Marcy & Britton, 2005; Bollini, Pampallona, Tibaldi, Kupelnick, & Munizza, 1999). Proposed medications such as clonidine, cyproheptadine, and benztropine (Marcy & Britton, 2005; Butt, 1989; Leemen, 1990) can cause dizziness as a side effect, which is unacceptable for patients with equilibrium disorders in addition to their hearing disorder. Protecting the hearing aid with a small plastic cover can be a solution in some cases; however, a hearing aid cannot operate in a vacuum.

THE IMPORTANCE OF CONSIDERING SIDE EFFECTS WHEN PRESCRIBING PSYCHOPHARMACOLOGICAL MEDICATION TO DEAF PATIENTS

The case histories mentioned in Tables 2 and 3 illustrate the important role side effects can play during the psychopharmacological treatment of deaf and hard of hearing patients. Physical, language, and communicative aspects related to the deafness can influence the treatment. The advantages of the treatment must be carefully weighed against the risks. Medication of patients coming from a "hearing" unit should be carefully screened on their value for the patient's mental disorder, their effectiveness, and possible side effects.

In view of all of these factors it is evident that psychopharmacological treatment should be tailored to the individual deaf patient (Landsberger & Diaz, 2010;

TABLE 3.   Increased Perspiration as a Side Effect of Antidepressant Medication and the Negative Consequences for Deaf and Hard of Hearing People

Patient Gender Age Origin	Profession	Type of Deafness	Hearing Aid	Mental disorder	Medication	Side effect after a few months/years	Consequences	Approach
1. Female 60 years Caucasian	Housewife	Hard of hearing, congenital	Hearing aid both sides	Chronic depressive disorder	Duloxetine 30 mg daily with sufficient effect	Excessive perspiration during work Naranja Probability Scale (PS) causal	Sound through hearing aid is muffled, as being underwater	Other medication: Bupropion, later same side effect
2. Male 50 years Caucasian	IT specialist	Progressive deafness and tinnitus at 20 years old	Hearing aid both sides	Chronic depressive disorder + suicidal ideation	Sertraline 50 mg daily with positive effect	Excessive perspiration during light exercise Naranja PS causal	Damage to hearing aid. Exercise without hearing aid difficult	Accepted side effect, because of positive effect of medication. Obtained special hearing aid.
3. Male 60 years Caucasian	Technician	Postlingual deaf due to encephalo-meningitis at 10 years old	Cochlear implant (CI)	Chronic depressive disorder	Paroxetine 20 mg daily moderate effect	Excessive perspiration always Naranja PS Scale causal	Short circuit in hearing aid of CI +electrical shock	Change of medication: Fluoxetine Side effect disappeared
4. Male 30 years Caucasian	Disabled benefits due to psychiatric disorder	Postlingual deaf due to encephalo-meningitis at 5 years old	None	Chronic Paranoid Schizophrenia with depressive symptoms	Olanzapine 15 mg daily Fluoxetine 20 mg daily Both sufficient effect	After 2 years: wet hands, arms, face and thorax increasingly in social meetings, Naranja PS causal	Avoids social situations and hand contact	Fluoxetine discontinued. Side effect disappeared, No relapse of depressive symptoms

Sleeboom-van Raaij, 1997; Sleeboom-van Raaij & Knoppert van der Klein, 2003). In addition to the effect of the medication itself, the side effects and the deaf patient's acceptance of them should determine the choice of drug (Sleeboom-van Raaij & Knoppert van der Klein, 2003).

Side effects are divided into three groups according to their severity and their negative impact on deaf and hard of hearing patients:

1. Unacceptable to deaf and hard of hearing patients
2. Unpleasant and often unacceptable to deaf and hard of hearing patients
3. Unpleasant but acceptable to deaf and hard of hearing patients

Use of Table 4, which lists unacceptable and unpleasant side effects in deaf and hard of hearing patients, in combination with a reliable psychopharmacological manual, may help avoid undesirable results.

Group 1: Unacceptable Side Effects

Tardive dyskinesia and extrapyramidal symptoms badly affect sign language expressively and motorially (Nobutomo & Inada, 2012; Advokat, Mayville, & Matson, 2000; Kamin et al., 2000). Visual disorders resulting from glaucoma and

TABLE 4.   Side Effects

1. Unacceptable Side Effects	2. Unpleasant and Often Unacceptable Side Effects	3. Unpleasant but Acceptable Side Effects
1. irreparable damage to the retina 2. irreversible movement disorder (tardive dyskinesia) 3. extreme extrapyramidal symptoms 4. glaucoma 5. tinnitus 6. disequilibrium 7. leukopenia 8. muscle weakness (hypotonia)	1. sedation 2. orthostatic hypotension (particularly in disequilibrium and visual impairment) 3. epileptogenic effect (especially in brain damage) 4. fatigue 5. increased perspiration	1. desirable or transient "sedation" 2. passing side effects 3. intestinal complaints 4. weight gain

damage to the retina hamper the understanding of sign language and, for late deaf and hard of hearing patients, also impede lipreading (Richa & Yazbek, 2010). The older, conventional antipsychotics and antidepressants can in fact cause glaucoma (ibid.). Loss of vision and equilibrium and the limitation of means of communication are problematic for everyone, but for deaf people who cannot compensate for these losses due to their deafness, these side effects can be quite traumatic. A decline in communication skills reduces opportunities for taking part in life within society and thus one's quality of life.

Tinnitus (a side effect of antidepressant medication) is very unpleasant for those who are (late) deaf and hard of hearing and can negatively influence the understanding of speech (Sleeboom-van Raaij, 2011; Langguth, Landgrebe, Wittmann, Kleinjung, & Hajak, 2010; Lareb, 2005). Deafness is often accompanied by vertigo; thus medication that causes disturbances of one's equilibrium can be very unpleasant for deaf patients (Trindade et al., 2008; Anderson, 2001). The negative effect of muscle weakness is illustrated in table 2.

Side effects can also have practical consequences. A traditional antipsychotic remedy, pimozide, had a positive influence on the tonicity of the musculature of a 50-year-old female patient with a rare, progressive, hereditary syndrome characterized by epilepsy, deafness, and ataxia. The patient was eventually able to sit upright.

Group 2: Unpleasant and Often Unacceptable Side Effects

The side effects mentioned in Group 2 are unpleasant and often unacceptable to deaf and hard of hearing patients. For example, eliciting epileptic fits or reducing reaction capabilities by sedation can be unacceptable in the workplace or while driving a vehicle. Fatigue and orthostatic hypotension are unpleasant but can be made bearable by following certain rules, such as taking regular breaks while working and sitting and getting up slowly (Figueroa, Basford, & Low, 2010; Trindade et al., 2008). Physical countermaneuvers involving isometrically contracting the muscles below the waist for about 30 seconds at a time can help to maintain blood pressure during daily activities (Figueroa et al., 2010).

Epilepsy can occur more often in patients with hereditary deafness and deafness resulting from brain damage. Prescribing epileptogenic medication such as certain antipsychotics and antidepressants can be hazardous to these patients. In this case extra alertness is necessary when one is taking a combination of medications in which the inhibition of the CYP450 enzymes' activity may increase the plasma concentration of the epileptogenic medication (Bootsma, 2004; Spina, 2002; Perucca, 2005; Sleeboom-van Raaij & Karmelk, 1999). Increased perspiration is explained in table 3.

Group 3: Unpleasant but Acceptable Side Effects

Group 3 comprises acceptable side effects. Sedation of a transient nature can require extra attention for deaf and hard of hearing individuals because it can negatively influence the alertness and concentration required for communication and safe practice. In general, there are several side effects that are unpleasant but acceptable or treatable for hearing as well as deaf patients (Kamin et al., 2000; Advokat et al., 2000; Trindade, 1998). It is important to be aware that deaf and hard of hearing patients should not experience limitations in their communicative abilities and social contacts.

Sometimes the unpleasant side effects of Groups 1 and 2 are unavoidable because no other pharmacological options are available. For example, if a psychotic patient does not accept oral administration of an antipsychotic medicine and the medication must be administered in a depot injection, then often the only antipsychotic medications remaining are the traditional ones, which have many side effects (Adam, Fenton, Quraishi, & David, 2001; Kamin et al., 2000).

RECOMMENDATIONS FOR THE PSYCHOPHARMACOLOGICAL TREATMENT OF DEAF PATIENTS

In general, the higher sensitivity to side effects, the limited language ability, and the increased risks because of physical disorders, can enhance the vulnerability of deaf and hard of hearing patients during the initiation of psychopharmacological medication. An individual plan has to be made, and side effects must be monitored. This can result in a long-term process to find the right medication (Sleeboom-van Raaij & Knoppert-van der Klein, 2003; du Feu & Fergusson, 2003). High-risk patients should be familiarized with possible side effects in a clinical inpatient service.

Antipsychotic Medication

Because of the higher incidence of EPS of the conventional antipsychotic agents compared to the atypical antipsychotics and the greater sensitivity of deaf patients to these side effects, as well as the impediments to communication and motor function they experience, it is advisable to choose the atypical antipsychotics and their injectable depot medication. This antipsychotic medication can—beside treating psychotic disorders—also be effective in behavioral disorders with aggression and paranoid behavior (Davison, 2005; Kamin et al., 2000; Buckley, 1999).

Antidepressive Medication

The physical symptoms of depression often make themselves felt first; it is therefore necessary to make a special effort to ask about any depressive feelings (Kapfhammer, 2006; Madhukar & Trivedi, 2004). A lack of expression of depressive feelings is caused by a poorly developed capacity to articulate one's emotions and the limited language and communication skills of many deaf patients (Landsberger & Diaz, 2010; Black & Glickman, 2006). Because of the side effects of tricyclic antidepressants, as mentioned in Groups 1 and 2, the use of SSRIs is advised. SSRIs have proven their efficacy in the treatment of aggression, impulse control disorders, compulsive disorders, phobias, anxiety, and panic disorders (Ables & Baughman, 2003; Schatzberg, 2000). Trazodone, a dicyclic antidepressant, has been proven effective as a sleep remedy without sedation by day in low dosages of 25–50 mg for antidepressant- or psychotropic-related insomnia (Kaynak, Kaynak, Gözükirmizi, & Guilleminault, 2004; Haffmans & Vos, 1999; Nierenberg, Adler, Peselow, Zornberg, & Rosenthal, 1994). The older tricyclic antidepressants are to be used only in cases of therapy-resistant depressions and, of this group, clomipramine in severe obsessive-compulsive disorders (Foa et al., 2005; Thorén, Asberg, Cronholm, Jörnestedt, & Träskman, 1988).

Antiepileptic Medication

The electroencephalogram of deaf patients with brain damage can display atypical nonepileptic abnormalities (Shelley, Trimble, & Boutros, 2008). The etiology of their deafness is often related to brain damage caused by meningoencephalitis, prenatal rubella or other prenatal infections, brain trauma, or similar conditions (Shelley et al., 2008; Pomeroy, Holmes, Dodge, & Feigin, 1990). Antiepileptic medications such as carbamazepine, valproate, and phenytoin can produce a clinical improvement in aggressiveness, agitation, impulsivity, and other behavioral and neurobehavioral disorders (Lane, Kjome, & Gerard Moeller, 2011; Huband, Ferriter, Nathan, & Jones, 2010).

Lithium

To date, the use of lithium has shown no particular side effects in treating deaf patients. However, lithium can have a negative effect on the functioning of the kidney and the thyroid gland. In case of comorbidity such as chronic renal failure in Alport's syndrome, BOR syndrome, Wolfram syndrome or other deafness-kidney syndromes and in hypothyroidism in Pendred's syndrome, lithium is best avoided, and other mood stabilizers such as carbamazepine and valproate should be the first drug of choice (Huang, Zdanski, & Castillo, 2012; Hildebrandt, 2010; Arwert & Sepers, 2008; Gorlin, Toriello, & Cohen, 1995).

Anxiolytics

Buspirone, when compared to diazepam and clorazepate, has been shown to have significantly less influence on psychomotor functioning and less of a sedative-hypnotic effect and to cause less lethargy (Newton, Casten, Alms, Benes, & Marunycz, 1982). For various patients suffering from hereditary syndromes such as cerebellar ataxia, this was useful during treatment and was effective in treating anxiety disorders.

Benzodiazepines with a long half-life and low potency (e.g., clorazepate and chlordiazepoxide) have proved to be the anxiolytics with the lowest tendency for abuse (Longo & Johnson, 2000). High-potency benzodiazepines, such as clonazepam, are prescribed for severe tinnitus. In a growing number of patients it has been shown to be an effective treatment, especially at night, when the tinnitus disturbed their sleep (Fornaro & Martino, 2010: Gananza 2002).

PSYCHOEDUCATION IN RELATION TO MENTAL DISORDERS AND MEDICATION

"Psychoeducation in its literal definition implies provision of information and education to a service user with severe and enduring mental illness including schizophrenia, about the diagnosis, the treatment, appropriate resources, prognosis, common coping strategies" (Pekkala & Merinder, 2002, p. 1). Psychoeducation is an important way to improve a patient's loyalty to treatment and therapy (Bäuml et al., 2006; Pekkala & Merinder, 2002). Interestingly, research on the best way to provide psychoeducation has shown that the way the psychoeducational intervention takes place is unimportant. Individual sessions, group therapy, or family therapy all have the same effect on the outcome of the treatment or relapse (Rummel-Kluge, Kluge, & Kissling, 2013). Although psychoeducation is offered mainly to patients with schizophrenia and depression, it is also effective for other mental health disorders such as bipolar disorder, anxiety, and dementia (ibid.).

Psychoeducation for deaf patients should be tailor-made, in other words adapted to their specific needs in communication and language (Landsberger & Diaz, 2010; Black & Glickman, 2006; du Feu & Fergusson, 2003; Sleeboom-van Raaij & Knoppert-van der Klein, 2003). Tamaskar et al. (2000) state that information to deaf individuals on health and preventive medicine had an effect only when the doctor provided this advice during an examination. Communication and cultural barriers should be overcome by the service by providing deaf staff members who work together with adequately trained medical professionals. This information would include the illness, the usefulness of the medication, the duration of the treatment, the possible results and side effects of the medication, and necessary interventions such as modifications to the patient's environment and regimen in relation to the syndrome (see Table 5).

TABLE 5.   Important Elements of Psychoeducation

I. Explaining	II. Necessary approach
1. the illness, • diagnosis • cause and background • course and prognosis • comorbidity • relation to the deafness and related factors 2. the usefulness and necessity of medication 3. effects and side effects of medication 4. treatment of side effects 5. the results of discontinuation of the medication 6. interaction with other medication 7. regimen to daily living: such as food, exercise, being outside, activities, work, alcohol 8. involvement of the family, • family support. • education of the family regarding the illness and the treatment. 9. Answering questions	1. tailor-made information for the patient with • adaptation of the language • adaptation of the communication • adaptation of the content of the information 2. note taking of the content of the session for the patient 3. relay interpreter 4. deaf staff 5. repeated sessions

Medical treatment must be a team effort involving the patient and the doctor, often in cooperation with the family and other professionals. This means that doctors must develop skills to enable deaf or hard of hearing patients to understand the issues; they must also be aware of the possible effects this knowledge may have on patients. Doctors must be prepared to adapt their course of action several times should the side effects cause problems. Nursing staff must be able to repeat the doctors' explanations and put these in writing for the patient.

Conversations require so much concentration for the deaf patient that making notes or remembering what has been said is at times not possible. Moreover, brochures about particular medications and mental illnesses are often written in inaccessible language and require clarification. Explanation of the medication is therefore an intensive process and must be repeated regularly (Sleeboom-van Raaij & Knoppert van der Klein, 2003). New information strategies and on the various aspects of psychiatric conditions and the importance of medical treatment and psychotherapy for deaf and hard of hearing patients and their families must be developed (Landsberger & Diaz, 2010; Black & Glickman, 2006; du Feu & Fergusson, 2003; Sleeboom-van Raaij & Knoppert-van der Klein, 2003).

The doctor-patient relationship, which should be a working alliance, thrives on the numerous consultations and can influence the patients' loyalty to therapy in a positive manner. The ultimate aim of psychoeducation must be the patients' acceptance of and adaptation to their illness and its treatment. In an ideal situation, patients and their relatives have acquired sufficient knowledge to cope with both the disorder and the treatment.

CONCLUSION

Deaf and hard of hearing people are normal people who, like hearing people, can acquire a mental illness. Psychiatric treatment may be necessary. In treating deaf patients, particular aspects relevant to deafness must be considered. The special needs of the deaf patient are connected to communication, language, emotional, developmental, medical, environmental, cultural, and social aspects. These special needs play an important role in the diagnostic and treatment process. Mental health professionals should be trained in these matters and their effect on diagnosis and treatment. Deaf staff members are necessary to overcome cultural and communication barriers and provide a deaf-friendly environment.

With respect to the pharmaceutical treatment of a mental illness in deaf and hard of hearing patients, it is important to be aware of their greater sensitivity to medication and the undesired and often serious side effects. A thorough knowledge of the application, effects, side effects, contraindications, and interactions with other medication is utterly essential. Careful and frequent explanation of the illness and treatment by mental health professionals who specialize in hearing impairment issues is also imperative. Finally, the treatment of deaf and hard of hearing patients should take place in a setting in which they are understood and their special needs are addressed. Only specialized mental health services for deaf and hard of hearing patients can provide this level of treatment.

REFERENCES

Ables, A. Z., & Baughman III, O. L. (2003). Antidepressants: Update on new agents and indications. *American Family Physician, 67,* 547–554.

Adam, S., Fenton, M. K. P., Quraishi, S., & David, A. S. (2001). Systematic meta-review of depot antipsychotic drugs for people with schizophrenia. *British Journal of Psychiatry, 179*, 290–299.

Advokat, C. D., Mayville, E. A., & Matson, J. L. (2000). Side effects profiles of atypical antipsychotics, typical antipsychotics, or no psychotropic medications in persons with mental retardation. *Research in Developmental Disabilities, 21*, 75–84.

Ammeyer, J. (2010). Congenital rubella syndrome and delayed manifestations. *International Journal of Pediatric Otorhinolaryngology, 74*, 1067–1070.

Anderson, I. M. (2001). Meta-analytical studies on new antidepressants. *British Medical Bulletin, 57*(1), 161–178.

Arwert, L. I., & Sepers, J. M. (2008). Goitre and hearing impairment in a patient with Pendred syndrome. *Netherlands Journal of Medicine, 66*(3), 118–120.

Banatvala, J. E., & Brown, D. W. G. (2004). Rubella. *Lancet, 363*(9415), 1127–1137.

Barnett, S. (2012). Long-term health implications of congenital rubella syndrome (CRS). Research project. London: Sense.

Basilier, T. (1973). Surdophrenia: The psychic consequences of congenital or early acquired deafness. Some theoretical and clinical considerations. *Acta Psychiatrica Scandinavica 40*(Suppl. 180), 362–374.

Bäuml, J., Fröböse, T., Kraemer, S., Rentrop, M., & Pitschel-Walz, G. (2006). Psychoeducation: A basic psychotherapeutic intervention for patients with schizophrenia and their families. *Schizophrenia Bulletin, 32*(Supp. 1), S1–S9.

Black, P. A., & Glickman, N. S. (2006). Demographics, psychiatric diagnoses, and other characteristics of North American deaf and hard-of-hearing inpatients. *Journal of Deaf Studies and Deaf Education 11* (3), 303–321.

Bollini, P., Pampallona, S., Tibaldi, G., Kupelnick, B., & Munizza, C. (1999). Effectiveness of antidepressants: Meta-analysis of dose-effect relationships in randomised clinical trials. *British Journal of Psychiatry 174*, 297–303.

Bootsma, H. P. R. (2004). Anti-epileptica en comedicatie: Handreikingen voor de praktijk. *Tijdschrift voor neurologie en neurochirurgie, 105*(1), 40–46.

Briffa, D. (1999). Deaf and mentally ill: Are their needs being met? *Australasian Psychiatry, 7*(1), 7–10.

Briffa, D. (2001). *Deafness and mental health: A report on the mental health needs of deaf and hearing impaired people in Queensland.* Brisbane: Queensland Government Health.

Brown A. S. (2011). Exposure to prenatal infection and risk of schizophrenia. *Frontiers in Psychiatry 2* (November), 1–5. doi:10.3389/fpsyt.2011.00063

Brown, A. S. (2012). Epidemiologic studies of exposure to prenatal infection and risk of schizophrenia and autism. *Developmental Neurobiology, 72*(10), 1272–1276.

Brown, A. S., Cohen, P., Harkavy-Friedman, J., Babulas, V., Malaspina, D., Gorman, J. M., et al. (2001). Prenatal rubella, premorbid abnormalities, and adult schizophrenia. *Biological Psychiatry, 49*, 473–486.

Brown, A. S., Schaefer, C. A., Quesenberry Jr., C. P., Liu, L., Babulas, V. P., & Susser, E. S. (2005). Maternal exposure to toxoplasmosis and risk of schizophrenia in adult offspring. *American Journal of Psychiatry, 162*, 767–773.

Buckley, P. F. (1999). The role of typical and atypical antipsychotic medications in the management of agitation and aggression. *Journal of Clinical Psychiatry, 60*(Suppl. 10), 52–60.

Buka, S. L., Tsuang, M. T., Torrey, E. F., Klebanoff, M. A., Bernstein, D., & Yolken, R. H. (2001). Maternal infections and subsequent psychosis among offspring. *Archives of General Psychiatry, 58*, 1032–1037.

Butt, M. M. (1989). Managing antidepressant-induced sweating [Letter]. *Journal of Clinical Psychiatry, 50,* 146–147.

Chaveiro, N., Celeno Porto, C., & Alves Barbosa, M. (2009). The relation between deaf patients and the doctor. *Revista Brasileira de Otorrinolaringologia, 75*(1), 147–150.

Chess, S., Korn, S., & Fernandez, P. (1971). *Psychiatric disorders of children with congenital rubella.* New York: Brunner/Mazel.

Davison, S. E. (2005). The management of violence in general psychiatry. *Advances in Psychiatric Treatment, 11,* 362–370.

Dammeyer J. (2010). Psychosocial development in a Danish population of children with cochlear implants and deaf and hard-of-hearing children. *Journal of Deaf Studies and Deaf Education. 15*(1), 50–58.

Denmark, J. C. (1994). *Deafness and mental health.* London: Jessica Kingsley Publishers.

Du Feu, M., & Fergusson, K. (2003). Sensory impairment and mental health. *Advances in Psychiatric Treatment, 9,* 95–103.

Duszak, R. S. (2009). Congenital rubella syndrome major review. *Optometry 80,* 36–43.

Ebert, D. A., & Heckerling, P. S. (1995). Communication with deaf patients: Knowledge, beliefs, and practices of physicians. *JAMA 273*(3), 227–229.

Fellinger, J., Holzinger, D., & Pollard, R. (2012). Mental health of deaf people. *Lancet, 379*(9820), 1037–1044.

Figueroa, J. J., Basford, J. R., & Low, P. A. (2010). Preventing and treating orthostatic hypotension: As easy as A, B, C. *Cleveland Clinic Journal of Medicine, 77*(5), 298–306.

Flexer, C. (1999). *Facilitating hearing and listening in young children* (2nd ed.). San Diego: Singular.

Foa, E. B., Liebowitz, M. R., Kozak, M. J., Sharon Davies, S., Campeas, R. M. D., Franklin, M. E., et al. (2005). Randomized, placebo-controlled trial of exposure and ritual prevention, clomipramine, and their combination in the treatment of obsessive-compulsive disorder. *American Journal of Psychiatry, 162*(1), 151–161.

Fornaro, M., & Martino, M. (2010). Tinnitus psychopharmacology: A comprehensive review of its pathomechanisms and management. *Neuropsychiatric Disease and Treatment, 6,* 209–218.

Ganança, M. M., Caovilla, H. H., Ganança, F. F., Ganança, C. F., Munhoz, M. S. L., Garcia da Silva, M. L., et al. (2002). Clonazepam in the pharmacological treatment of vertigo and tinnitus. *International Tinnitus Journal, 8*(1), 50–53.

Gorlin, R. J., Toriello, H. V., & Cohen, M. M. (1995). *Hereditary hearing loss and its syndromes.* New York: Oxford University Press.

Haffmans, P. M., & Vos, M. S. (1999). The effects of trazodone on sleep disturbances induced by brofaromine. *European Psychiatry, 14*(3), 167–171.

Haskins, B. G. (2004). Serving deaf adult psychiatric inpatients. *Psychiatric Services, 55*(5), 439–441.

Hildebrandt, F. (2010). Renal medicine 1: Genetic kidney diseases. *Lancet, 375,* 1287–1295.

Hindley, P., & Kitson, N. (Eds.). (2000). *Mental health and deafness.* London: Whurr.

Hindley, P., & van Gent, T. (2002). Psychiatric aspects of sensory impairments. In M. Rutter & E. Taylor (Eds.), *Child and adolescent psychiatry* (4th ed., 842–857). London: Blackwell.

Huang, B. Y., Zdanski, C., & Castillo, M. (2012). Pediatric sensorineural hearing loss. Part 2: Syndromic and acquired causes. *American Journal of Neuroradiology, 33,* 399–406.

Huband, N., Ferriter, M., Nathan, R., & Jones, H. (2010, February 17). Epileptics for aggression and associated impulsivity. *Cochrane Database Systemic Review 2,* CD003499. doi: 10.1002/14651858.CD003499.pub3

Jyonouchi, S., McDonald-McGinn, D. M., Bale, S., Zackai, E. H., & Sullivan, K. E. (2009). CHARGE (coloboma, heart defect, choanal atresia, retarded growth and development, genital hypoplasia, ear anomalies/deafness) syndrome and chromosome 22q11.2 deletion syndrome: A comparison of immunologic and nonimmunologic phenotypic features. *Pediatrics, 123*(5), e871–e877.

Kalachnik, J. E. (1988). Medication monitoring procedures: Thou shall, here's how. In K. D. Gadow & A. C. Poling (Eds.), *Pharmacotherapy and mental retardation* (pp. 231–232). Boston: Little, Brown.

Kalachnik, J. E. (1999). Measuring side effects of psychopharmacologic medication in individuals with mental retardation and developmental disabilities. *Mental Retardation and Developmental Disabilities Research Reviews, 5,* 348–359.

Kamin, J., Manwani, S., & Hughes, D. (2000). Extrapyramidal side effects in the psychiatric emergency service. *Psychiatric Services, 51*(3), 287–289.

Kapfhammer, H.-P. (2006). Somatic symptoms in depression. *Dialogues in Clinical Neuroscience, 8*(2), 227–239.

Kaynak, H., Kaynak, D., Gözükirmizi, E., & Guilleminault, C. (2004). The effects of trazodone on sleep in patients treated with stimulant antidepressants. *Sleep Medicine, 5*(1), 15–20.

Korkeila, J., Salokangas, R. K. R., Heinimaaa, M., Svirskis, T., Laine, T., Ruhrmann, S., et al. (2013). Physical illnesses, developmental risk factors, and psychiatric diagnoses among subjects at risk of psychosis. *European Psychiatry, 28*(3), 135–140.

Kulthanan, K., Jiamton, S., Boochangkool, K., & Jongjarearnprasert, K. (2007). Clinical study: Angioedema: Clinical and etiological aspects. *Clinical and Developmental Immunology,* article ID 26438.

Landsberger, S., & Diaz, D. R. (2010). Inpatient psychiatric treatment of deaf adults: Demographic and diagnostic comparisons with hearing inpatients' psychiatric services. *Psychiatric Services, 61*(2), 196–199.

Lane, C. D., Kjome, K. L., & Gerard Moeller, F. G. (2011). Neuropsychiatry of aggression. *Neurologic Clinics, 29*(1), 49–64.

Langguth, B., Landgrebe, M., Wittmann, M., Kleinjung, T., & Hajak, G. (2010, August). Persistent tinnitus induced by tricyclic antidepressants. *Journal of Psychopharmacology, 24*(8), 1273–1275.

Lareb. (2005). *SSRIs en tinnitus.* Den Bosch, the Netherlands: Lareb.

Leeman, C. P. (1990). Pathophysiology of tricyclic-induced sweating. *Journal of Clinical Psychiatry, 51,* 258–259.

Lezzoni, L. L., O'Day, B. L., Killeen, M., & Harker, H. (2004). Communicating about health care: Observations from persons who are deaf or hard of hearing. *Annals of Internal Medicine, 140*(5), 356–362. www.annals.org

Lin, C.-E., & Chen, C.-L. (2010). Case report: Repeated angioedema following administration of venlafaxine and mirtazapine. *General Hospital Psychiatry, 32,* 341.e1–341.e2.

Lingjærde, O., Ahlfors, U. G., Bech, P., Dencker, S. J., & Elgen, K. (1987). The UKU side effect rating scale: A new comprehensive rating scale for psychotropic drugs and a cross-sectional study of side effects in neuroleptic-treated patients. *Acta Psychiatrica Scandinavica, 76*(Suppl. 334), 1–100.

Longo, L. P., & Johnson, B. (2000, April 1). Addiction: Part I. Benzodiazepines—side effects, abuse risk and alternatives. *American Family Physician, 61*(7), 2121–2128.

Madhukar, H., & Trivedi, M. D. (2004). The link between depression and physical symptoms. *Primary Care Companion Journal of Clinical Psychiatry 6*(Suppl. 1), 12–16.

Mago, R., & Monti, D. (2007). Antiadrenergic treatment of antidepressant-induced excessive sweating in 3 patients. *Journal of Clinical Psychiatry, 68,* 639–640.

Mago, R., Thase, M. E., & Rovner, B. W. (2013, May 1). Antidepressant-induced excessive sweating: Clinical features and treatment with terazosin. *Annals of Clinical Psychiatry, 25*(2), E1–E7.

Marcy, T. R., & Britton, M. L. (2005). Antidepressant-induced sweating. *Annals of Pharmacotherapy., 39,* 748–752.

Moleman, P., & Birkenhäger, W. H. (2008). *Praktische psychofarmacologie.* Prelum Uitgevers: Houten, the Netherlands.

Munro, L., Knox, M., & Lowe, R. (2008). Exploring the potential of constructionist therapy: Deaf clients, hearing therapists and a reflecting team. *Journal of Deaf Studies and Deaf Education, 13*(3), 307–323.

Naranjo, C. A., Busto, U., Sellers, E. M., Sandor, P., Ruiz, I., Roberts, E. A., et al. (1981). A method for estimating the probability of adverse drug reactions. *Clinical Pharmacology and Therapeutics 30,* 239–245.

Newton, R. E., Casten, G. P., Alms, D. R., Benes, C. O., & Marunycz, J. D. (1982). The side effect profile of buspirone in comparison to active controls and placebo. *Journal of Clinical Psychiatry, 43*(12, Part 2), 100–102.

Nierenberg, A. A., Adler, L. A., Peselow, E., Zornberg, G., & Rosenthal, M. (1994). Trazodone for antidepressant-associated insomnia. *American Journal of Psychiatry, 151*(7), 1069–1072.

Nobutomo, Y., & Inada, T. (2012). Dystonia secondary to use of antipsychotic agents. In R. Rosales (Ed.), *Dystonia: The many facets* (pp. 55–64). Rijeka, Croatia: InTech Europe.

O'Donnell, N. (1991). *A report on a survey of late emerging manifestations of congenital rubella syndrome.* New York: Helen Keller National Center.

Pekkala, E., & Merinder, L. (2002). Psychoeducation for schizophrenia. *Cochrane Database Systemic Review.* CD002831.

Pereira, P. C., & Fortes, P. A. (2010). Communication and information barriers to health assistance for deaf patients. *American Annals of the Deaf, 155*(1), 31–37.

Perucca, E. (2005). Clinically relevant drug interactions with antiepileptic drugs. *British Journal of Clinical Pharmacology, 61*(3), 246–255.

Pisani, F., Oteri, G., Costa, C., Di Raimondo, G., & Di Perri, R. (2002). Effects of psychotropic drugs on seizure threshold. *Drug Safety, 25*(2), 91–110.

Pomeroy, S. L., Holmes, S. J., Dodge, P. R., & Feigin, R. D. (1990). Seizures and other neurologic sequelae of bacterial meningitis in children. *New England Journal of Medicine, 323,* 1651–1657.

Queensland Health. (2008). *Deafness and mental health: Guidelines for working with persons who are deaf or hard of hearing.* Brisbane, Australia: Princess Alexandra Hospital Health Service District.

Rainer, J. D., & Altshuler, K. Z. (1966). *Comprehensive mental health services for the deaf.* New York: New York State Psychiatric Institute, Department of Medical Genetics, Columbia University.

Remvig, J. (1969). Deaf mutism and psychiatry. *Acta Psychiatrica Scandinavica, 36*(Suppl. 210), 9–120.

Reznik, I., Volchek, L., Mester, R., Kotler, M., Sarova-Pinhas, I., Spivak, B., et al. (2000, September–October). Myotoxicity and neurotoxicity during clozapine treatment. *Clinical Neuropharmacology, 23*(5), 276–280.

Richa, S., & Yazbek, J. C. (2010). Ocular adverse effects of common psychotropic agents: A review. *Central Nervous System Drugs, 24*(6), 501–526.

Ruffmann, C., Bogliun, G., & Beghi, E. (2006, April). Epileptogenic drugs: A systematic review. *Expert Review Neurotherapeutics, 6*(4), 575–689.

Rummel-Kluge, C., Kluge, M., & Kissling, W. (2013). Frequency and relevance of psycho-education in psychiatric diagnoses: Results of two surveys five years apart in German-speaking European countries. *BMC Psychiatry, 13,* 170.

Schatzberg, A. F. (2000). New indications for antidepressants. *Journal of Clinical Psychiatry, 61*(Supplement. 11), 9–17.

Scheier, D. B. (2009, Spring–Summer). Barriers to health care for people with hearing loss: A review of the literature. *Journal New York State Nurses Association, 40*(1), 4–10.

Shelley, B. P., Trimble, M. R., & Boutros, N. N. (2008). Electroencephalographic cerebral dysrhythmic abnormalities in the trinity of nonepileptic general population, neuropsychiatric, and neurobehavioral disorders. *Journal of Neuropsychiatry and Clinical Neurosciences, 20,* 7–22.

Shinohara, Y. (2009, April). Excessive sweating in a male patient caused by milnacipran. *Indian J Psychiatry, 51*(2), 162.

Sleeboom-van Raaij, C. J. (1991). Issues of importance to be considered in setting up new mental health services for the deaf. In Luc Walraedt (Ed.), *Proceedings of the Second International Congress of the European Society for Mental Health and Deafness* (pp. 139–143). Namur, Belgium: La Bastide and the European Society Mental Health and Deafness.

Sleeboom-van Raaij, C. J. (1997). *Psycho-pharmacological treatment and deafness: Hazards and highlights.* Paper presented at the Fourth International Congress of the European Society for Mental Health and Deafness, Manchester.

Sleeboom-van Raaij, C. J. (1999). Zichtbaar anders: De visuele interactie afdeling Nederlands. *Tijdschrift voor Medische Administratie,* 5–7.

Sleeboom-van Raaij, C. J. (2000). Màs allá del período pionero. In T. Orihuela (Ed.), *Salud mental y sordera* (pp. 209–221). Zamora, Spain: Edintras.

Sleeboom-van Raaij, C. J. (2008). Psychofarmaca bij de psychiatrische behandeling van doven en slechthorenden. *Psyfar,* 40–43.

Sleeboom-van Raaij, C. J. (2010). Overmatige transpiratie bij antidepressiva. *Psyfar, 3,* 38–41.

Sleeboom-van Raaij, C. J. (2011). De rol van psychofarmaca bij de behandeling van tinnitus. *Psyfar, 2,* 54–57.

Sleeboom-van Raaij, C. J., & Karmelk, F. (1999, January–February). Antipsychotica bij een epilepsiepatiënt. *Janssen-Cilag Medisch Wetenschappelijk Nieuws,* 14–15.

Sleeboom-van Raaij, C. J., & Knoppert van der Klein, E. A. M. (2003). Complicerende factoren in de psychiatrische behandeling van doven en slechthorenden. In A. Bakker & A. Korzec (Eds.), *De gecompliceerde kliniek 2003: Als protocollen en richtlijnen tekortschieten* (pp. 78–85). Amsterdam: Benecke.

Spina, E., & Perucca, E. (2002). Clinical significance of pharmacokinetic interactions between antiepileptic and psychotropic drugs. *Epilepsia, 43*(Suppl. 2), 37–44.

Steinberg, A. G. (1991). Issues in providing mental health services to hearing-impaired persons. *Hospital & Community Psychiatry, 42*(4), 380–389.

Steinberg, A. G., Barnett, S., Meador, H. E., Wiggins, E. A., & Zazove, P. (2006). Healthcare system accessibility: Experiences and perceptions of deaf people. *Journal of General Internal Medicine, 21,* 260–266.

Steinberg, A. G., Sullivan, V. J., & Loew, R. C. (1998). Cultural and linguistic barriers to mental health service access: The deaf consumer's perspective. *American Journal of Psychiatry, 155,* 982–984.

Steinberg, A. G., Wiggins, E. A., Barmada, C. H., and Sullivan, V. J. (2002). Deaf women: experiences and perceptions of healthcare system access. *Journal of Women's Health 11*(8), 729–741.

Tamaskar, P., Malia, T., Stern, C., Gorenflo, D., Meador, H., & Zazove, P. (2000, June). Preventive attitudes and beliefs of deaf and hard-of-hearing individuals. *Archives of Family Medicine., 9*(6), 518–525, discussion 526.

Thorén, P., Asberg, M., Cronholm, B., Jörnestedt, L., & Träskman, L. (1980). Clomipramine treatment of obsessive-compulsive disorder. Part I: A controlled clinical trial. *Archives of General Psychiatry, 37*(11), 1281–1285.

Trindade, E., Menon, D., Topfer, L. A., & Coloma, C. (2008). Adverse effects associated with selective serotonin reuptake inhibitors and tricyclic antidepressants: A meta-analysis. *Canadian Medical Association Journal, 159,* 1245–1252.

Vancampfort, D., Probst, M., De Herdt, A., Nunes, R. M., Corredeira, M., Carraro, A., Wachter, D. D., & De Hert, M. (2013). An impaired health related muscular fitness contributes to a reduced walking capacity in patients with schizophrenia: a cross-sectional study. *BMC Psychiatry, 13,* 5.

van Gent, T. (2012). *Mental health problems in deaf and severely hard of hearing children and adolescents: Findings on prevalence, pathogenesis and clinical complexities, and implications for prevention, diagnosis and intervention.* Doctoral dissertation, Leiden University. Leiden: Drukkerij Mostert.

van Harten, P. N. (1998). Movement disorders associated with neuroleptics. Unpublished doctoral dissertation, University of Utrecht, Utrecht.

van Harten, P. N. (2000). *Bewegingsstoornissen door antipsychotica.* Amsterdam: Boom.

Van Nunen-Schrauwen, T., & Schoenmaker, A. (2007). Medical and psychological impact of congenital rubella syndrome in adults. In S. Munore (Ed.), *Proceedings of the 14th Deafblind International World Conference, September 25–30, Perth, Australia.* Burswood, Australia: DeafBlind International.

Waddell, L., & Taylor, M. (2008). A new self-rating scale for detecting atypical or second-generation antipsychotic side effects. *Journal of Psychopharmacology, 22,* 238–243.

Zazove, P., Niemann, L. C., Gorenflo, D. W., Carmack, C., Mehr, D., Coyne, J. C., et al. (1993). The health status and health care utilization of deaf and hard-of-hearing persons. *Archives Family Medicine, 2*(7), 745–752.

3

Mental Health Services in Mexico: Challenges and Proposals

Benito Estrada Aranda

WHY PROVIDE SPECIALIZED MENTAL HEALTH SERVICES TO DEAF PERSONS?

In England, collaboration between the National Institute of Mental Health and the Health Department resulted in a publication titled *Mental Health and Deafness: Toward Equity and Access: Best Practice Guidance* (NIMHE/DH, 2005). Their data show significant relationships between mental disorders and deafness. For example, 40% of deaf children are described as having behavior disorders, compared with 25% of hearing children. Studies carried out in different countries have indicated relatively higher levels of mental disorders and alcohol problems in deaf adults. Hypotheses about these data address the likelihood of brain damage at birth, as well as the effects of social exclusion (Estrada, 2008), including limited opportunities for education and employment. Contributing to this social exclusion is the use of a sign language, which is marginal, visual, and unfamiliar to hearing persons, including those hearing families with deaf children. This situation applies to about 90% of deaf and hard of hearing individuals.

In Mexico, with a population of about 112 million (INEGI, 2010), only about 2% of the annual health budget, which itself averages about 6.5% annually, is assigned to public mental health services for the country, according to data compiled by the World Health Organization (WHO), the Pan-American Health Organization, and the Mexico Ministry of Health (IESM-OMS, 2011), working in collaboration. Of that 2%, about 80% is used to cover the expenses of inpatient psychiatric hospitals. No public mental health services for deaf and hard of hearing people (i.e., with sign language accessibility) are either mentioned or currently available. It should be noted that WHO recommends that about 10% of a national health budget should be devoted to mental health, yet the average mental health budget for medium- to high-income countries is only about 2% (WHO, 2004), thus putting Mexico below average.

In addition to the lack of services for deaf and hard of hearing people in Mexico, there are shortages of these services to the general population as well. According to the report mentioned earlier, the total number of mental health service providers is about 10,000 persons, with approximately 1.6 psychiatrists, 1 physician, 3 nurses, 1 psychologist, 0.5 social workers, 0.19 therapists, and 2 health professionals/ technicians per 100,000 inhabitants, with most inadequately distributed throughout the population and concentrated primarily in psychiatric hospitals.

The following discussion reviews the problems and challenges of providing mental health services to Deaf people and then sets out several proposals for establishing such services. In this chapter, "Deaf" (with a capital *D*) refers to people who are congenitally and/or prelingually deaf and consider themselves part of Deaf culture and the Deaf community, which predominantly uses Mexican Sign Language (MSL).

Demographic Issues of the Mexican Deaf Population

Approximately 1 or 2 out of 1,000 individuals around the world are born severely or profoundly deaf (ADSS, BDA, LGA, NCB, NDCS, & RNID, 2002). Although in 2001 the World Health Organization estimated that about 250 million people have a hearing disability, it is still difficult to obtain more specific data from most countries.

Although Mexico does not have an official or a specific census of deaf individuals, extrapolations from the last two population censuses suggest an increase of nearly double that number. The XII General Census of Population and Dwelling (INEGI, 2000) indicated almost three individuals with a hearing disability for every 1,000 inhabitants in the country, or a total of 281,000, with about 31.2% residing in rural areas. In 2010, the XIII General Census of Population and Dwelling (INEGI, 2010) indicated a total of 498,640 people with a hearing disability (273,216 males and 225,424 females). In 10 years, just about double the number of individuals with a hearing disability were identified, the majority of whom were male (INEGI, 2000). Also noted was considerable variation in the distribution of individuals with a hearing disability throughout the country: 57,792 persons counted in the State of Mexico; 45,429 in the Distrito Federal; 37,662 in the State of Veracruz; 29,960 in the State of Jalisco; 14,192 in Nuevo León; and 2,230 in the State of Baja California Sur (ibid.).

It should also be noted that the definition of hearing disability is quite broad: "a loss or restriction of the ability to receive verbal or other audible messages" (Estrada, 2008) and thus does not reflect the heterogeneity of hearing impairment (Fellinger, Holzinger, & Pollard, 2012). Given the need to know how many of these individuals have inherited or acquired deafness, prelingually (prior to age 3) or postlingually, it is difficult to formulate appropriate mental health policies and services.

In terms of access to general health services, fewer than 50% of Deaf people overall (and in rural areas even fewer) can obtain these. Of those who have access to health care, 71.8% are recipients of Mexican Institute of Social Security (IMSS) services; 13.4% use the Institute of Security and Social Welfare Services of State Workers (ISSTE), while 8.7% have been assisted in private consultation (INEGI, 2004). These figures suggest some violation of human rights to health protection, as recognized by the National Commission of Human Rights (CNDH), as well as some noncompliance with Article 7 of Mexico's General Law on Persons with Disabilities, which was passed in 2005.

In Mexico, people have access to a free mental health public services network, but unfortunately none of these free services have specialized professionals who know sign language and understand Deaf culture. This situation presents a hardship for Deaf people in Mexico since evidence shows that Deaf people may experience mental illnesses and some psychological disorders more frequently than do hearing people (Estrada, Delgado, & Beyebach, 2010; Estrada & Ruiz, 2012; Leigh et al., 1989; Marcus, 1991; McGhee, 1995; Watt & Davis, 1991; Leigh & Anthony, 2001). Some studies have found a depression profile characterized by more somatic, cognitive, affective, and motivational symptoms in Deaf persons (Estrada, 2008; Estrada & Ruiz, 2012; Sanz, Navarro, & Vázquez, 2003; Beck, Steer, & Brawn, 1996). Another difference is that both Deaf men and women report depression symptoms with equal frequency (Estrada, 2008; Estrada & Ruiz, 2012), whereas among hearing people, women report depression more frequently than men.

Other studies indicate that Deaf children are more vulnerable to mental health problems than hearing children (National Institute for Mental Health in England/Department of Health, 2003), and behavioral disorders appear at least twice as frequently in Deaf children than in hearing ones (Meadow, 1981; Hindley et al., 1994; British Society for Mental Health and Deafness, 1998). Deaf children are also more vulnerable to physical, emotional, and sexual abuse than hearing children (ADSS et al., 2001) and exhibit more retardation or delay in their academic and psychosocial development, as well as increased frustration with regard to comprehension or cognition difficulties (Denmark, 1994).

By contrast, Deaf children of Deaf parents (around 10% of the Deaf population) tend to have better academic and more self-esteem than do Deaf children of hearing parents (Health Advisory Service, 1996). This is largely attributable to the relative ease with which the former acquire (sign) language and the challenge the latter face in obtaining any language, signed or spoken.

With respect to the education of Deaf people in Mexico, access to bilingual education or health services—without communication barriers—is still significantly lacking (Estrada, 2008). Deaf people are considered a vulnerable group by the National Commission on Human Rights (CNDH, 2008). According to INEGI (2004) data, more than half of Mexico's Deaf population does not go to school. On average, most Deaf people obtain about 3.4 years of schooling. Only 4.4% of this population has more than an intermediate-level education; 3.0% attend a university as undergraduates; and 0.2% have a master's degree or a doctorate. Coincidentally, around half of Mexico's Deaf population earns an inadequate income from employment.

Although sign language has been recognized as an official language by the Mexican government since about 2005, there are still insufficient numbers of signing Deaf people or sign language interpreters to provide full accessibility to education, health, or legal services, among other things. Due to these continuing barriers, Deaf people in Mexico continue to be at risk of significant social exclusion.

Challenges

While mental health services continue to be insufficient for the general hearing population, they continue to be almost nonexistent for Deaf people. A critical need exists for mental health professionals to receive specialized training in sign language, diagnosis, and treatment of Deaf people. Additionally, Deaf people often need more support services in the mental health system than do hearing people (Sleeboom, 1994, 2000; see also chapter 1 in this book). The main challenge is for mental health to become more of a priority in the national budget in general and thus to provide additional resources to reduce the disparity between the services available to Deaf and hearing people.

In addition to the obvious need for sign language and communication skills, mental health professionals who specialize in the treatment of Deaf people also need training in several other areas (Sleeboom, 2000), including etiology and onset of deafness, language issues, and other unique psychosocial and developmental matters.

Compounding the issues inherent in a lack of trained specialized mental health professionals is the fact that many Deaf people do not even understand what mental health services are. For example, they have no knowledge of the kinds of services a psychologist or psychiatrist offers or the differences between the various mental health services, such as substance abuse, family therapy, psychosocial rehabilitation, domestic violence, and sexual abuse. For this reason, such services for Deaf people in Mexico will need to start with accessible outreach and education campaigns.

To promote and establish mental health services for Deaf people in Mexico, the National Institute for Mental Health in England and the Department of Health (2005) propose the following:

1. Starting with the States of the Republic that have the highest numbers of Deaf people, conduct surveys to determine the mental health needs of Deaf individuals and where they are located. This will help identify the most likely accessible locations for these specialized services. Deaf people also need access to

the continuum of mental health services, ranging from ambulatory to inpatient psychiatric.

2. Conduct epidemiological studies with strong methodology to evaluate the incidence and prevalence of mental health issues in the Mexican Deaf population.

3. Increase the number of specialized mental health professionals trained to work with Deaf people. Since MSL is an officially recognized language in Mexico, the mental health network needs to include training of personnel in hospitals and clinics, as well as offer services by professionals who are themselves Deaf and/or fluent in sign language. Given that so few Deaf people are in graduate training programs, this goal may take longer to achieve.

4. Because the Mexican Deaf community is diverse and heterogeneous, as are other types of minority groups, mental health services for Deaf people should collaborate with the various Deaf organizations around the country, respecting the cultural and language variations involved. Additionally, mental health services should address the needs of Deaf-Blind individuals as well as Deaf people with other additional disabilities.

5. Mental health services need to be made as barrier-free as possible. That will include not only architectural but also technological modifications, such as text telephones, and visual emergency alarms and alerts. Ideally, mental health professionals who are themselves fluent in sign language should be hired; however, there will still be a need for sign language interpreters who are skilled in the mental health field. Currently no such training is available for this in Mexico.

Current Developments

Despite the establishment of the General Law on Persons with Disabilities (2005) and the more recent General Law for the Inclusion of Persons with Disabilities (2011) in Mexico, progress has been slow. It was not until 2010 that the first medical service accessible to Deaf people was established at the Mexican Institute of Social Security in the city of Tijuana. In addition to a Deaf physician, the service also has hearing physicians, nurses, and social welfare workers with Mexican Sign Language skills.

Also in 2010 the National Council for Persons with Disabilities (CONADIS) began certifying MSL interpreters, so that a greater number of qualified interpreters will be available to Deaf people in all public services. This will mean an increased need for professional and graduate study programs for people who want to become certified interpreters.

Prior to the Fifth World Congress on Mental Health and Deafness, organized by the Universidad Autónoma de Nuevo León and its College of Psychology and held in the city of Monterrey in May 2012, there was almost no opportunity for an exchange of academic research findings on mental health issues related to

Deaf people. This congress represented an opportunity to review and analyze the importance of promoting mental health and deafness services in Mexico.

CONCLUSIONS

Despite the existence of several new laws in Mexico, as discussed earlier, the development of mental health services for Deaf people has been very slow. The dearth of demographic and epidemiological information about the Deaf population in Mexico, their lack of access to education and other public services, inadequate employment opportunities for these individuals, and insufficient advocacy have kept this population from being visible. The Fifth World Congress on Mental Health and Deafness, held in Mexico in 2012, has done much to bring these issues to the forefront and hopefully will accelerate the expansion of services for this population.

REFERENCES

Association of Directors of Social Services (ADSS), British Deaf Association (BDA), Local Government Association (LGA), National Children's Bureau (NCB), National Deaf Children's Society (NDCS), & Royal National Institute for Deaf People (RNID). (2002). *Deaf children: Positive practice standards in social services.* London: RNID.

Beck, A. T., Steer, R. A., & Brown, G. K. (1996). *Manual for the Beck Depression Inventory-II.* San Antonio, TX: Psychological Corporation.

British Society for Mental Health and Deafness (BSMHD). (1998). *Forging new channels: Commissioning and delivering mental health services for people who are deaf: An NHS health advisory service thematic review.* Beaconsfield, Buckinghamshire, UK: BSMHD.

Comisión Nacional de Derechos Humanos (CNDH). (2008). Los derechos humanos de las personas con discapacidad auditiva. Available from http://www.cndh.org.mx.

Denmark, J. C. (1994). *Deafness and mental health.* London: Kingsley.

Estrada, A. B. (2008). La vulneración de los derechos humanos de las personas sordas en México. *Revista del Centro Nacional de Derechos Humanos, 3*(8), 105–127.

Estrada, A. B., Delgado, C., & Beyebach, M. (2010). Beck Depression Inventory-II in Spanish Sign Language. *International Journal of Hispanic Psychology, 3*(1), 25–46.

Estrada, A. B., & Ruiz, I. R. (2012, October). Beck Depression Inventory-II in Mexican Sign Language. *International Journal of Mental Health and Deafness, 2*(1). Available from www.ijmhd.org.

Fellinger, J., Holzinger, D., & Pollard, R. (2012). Mental health of deaf people. *Lancet, 379,* 1037–1044.

Health Advisory Service. (1996). *Mental health services: Forging new channels (Commissioning and delivering mental health services for people who are deaf).* London: BSMHD.

Hindley, P., Hill, P., McGuigan, S., & Kitson, N. (1994). Psychiatric disorders in deaf and hearing impaired children and young people: A prevalence study. *Journal of Child Psychology and Psychiatry, 55,* 917–934.

IESM-OMS. (2011). *Informe sobre sistema de salud mental en México.*

INEGI. (2000). *XII Censo general de población y vivienda 2000.*

INEGI. (2004). *Las personas con discapacidad en México: Una visión censal.*

INEGI. (2010). *XIII Censo general de población y vivienda 2010.*

Leigh, I. W., & Anthony, S. (2001). Reliability of the BDI-II with deaf persons. *Rehabilitation Psychology, 46*(2), 195–202.

Leigh, I. W., Robins, C. J., Welkowitz, J., & Bond, R. (1989). Toward greater understanding of depression in deaf individuals. *American Annals of the Deaf, 134,* 249–254.

Marcus, A. L. (1991). The prevalence of depression among deaf college students. Unpublished doctoral dissertation, Temple University, Philadelphia.

McGhee, H. (1995). An evaluation of modified written and American Sign Language versions of the Beck Depression Inventory with the prelingually deaf. Unpublished doctoral dissertation, California School of Professional Psychology, Alameda.

Meadow, K. (1981). Studies of behaviour problems of deaf children. In L. Stein, E. Mindel., & T. Jabaley (Eds.), *Deafness and mental health* (pp. 3–22). New York: Grune and Stratton.

National Institute for Mental Health in England/Department of Health (NIMHE/DH). (2003). *A sign of the times: Modernising mental health services for people who are deaf.* London: BSMHD.

National Institute for Mental Health in England/Department of Health (NIMHE/DH). (2005). *Mental health and deafness: Towards Equity and Access.* Leeds: Department of Health.

Orihuela, T., Conde, R., Vargas, M., Martínez, M. J., & Franco, M. A. (2000). Consideraciones preliminares al concepto de salud mental. In T. Orihuela (Ed.), *Salud mental y sordera* (pp. 35–79). Zamora: Edintras.

Sanz, J., Navarro, M., & Vázquez, C. (2003). Adaptación española del inventario para la depresión de Beck-II (BDI-II): 1. Propiedades psicométricas en estudiantes universitarios. *Análisis y modificación de conducta, 29*(124), 239–288.

Sleeboom, V. I. (1994). Differences in the treatment of deaf and hearing patients. In *Proceedings of the Third International Congress of the European Society for Mental Health and Deafness: Deafness and well-being: Contributions of deaf and hard of hearing professionals to the improvement of mental health and deafness practice* (pp. 75–76). Paris: Éditions Charles Léopold Mayer.

Sleeboom, V. I. (2000). Más allá del período pionero. In T. Orihuela (Ed.), *Salud mental y sordera* (pp. 209–221). Zamora: Edintras.

Watt, J. D., & Davis, F. E. (1991). The prevalence of boredom proneness and depression among profoundly deaf residential school adolescents. *American Annals of the Deaf, 136,* 409–413.

World Health Organization (WHO). (2004). *Invertir en salud mental.* Geneva: Organización Mundial de la Salud.

4

Eye Movement Desensitization and Reprocessing (EMDR) in Family Systems with Deaf Family Members

Lieke Doornkate

Deaf people, as well as their family members, have higher than average rates of mental health problems (Fellinger, Holzinger, & Pollard, 2012; Schultz Myers, Myers, & Marcus, 1999). An inability to hear can lead to social limitations, stigmatization, and impairments in emotional development. As a result, more deaf and hard of hearing people experience psychopathology than hearing people. In addition, numerous unique, trauma-type experiences appear in deaf adults: an average of 6.18 per person (SD = 2.65) (Schild & Dalenberg, 2012).

Eye movement desensitization and reprocessing (EMDR) is a promising technique that addresses the consequences of posttraumatic stress disorder (PTSD) in this group of clients. The method is partly nonverbal and therefore compatible with the visual world of deaf and hard of hearing people. EMDR is a protocol-based method for treating PTSD. It has been empirically validated for adult PTSD and is now administered successfully to hearing adults. Children also appear to benefit from EMDR.

EMDR

Originated by U.S. psychologist Francine Shapiro in 1989 and used as part of a more comprehensive course of therapy, EMDR, as already mentioned, is considered effective in treating PTSD and trauma-related anxiety disorders. Lauded for its efficiency, as it often produces desired results in one or a few sessions, the method has been empirically validated in use with traumatized adults and children. It has also been used in the treatment of more complex traumas and syndromes. The underlying theory of EMDR assumes that the natural healing process has been stymied by the tremendous amount of cognitive, visual, and emotional information generated by a traumatic event. If dysfunctional meanings are attached to such information as it is stored, PTSD symptoms occur (van der Kolk 1996; Shapiro, 2001). Using the more streamlined EMDR approach, clients often report reductions of debilitating symptoms such as reexperiencing (or reliving), nightmares, irritability, and extreme avoidance behavior.

Various explanations have been advanced for the therapeutic action of EMDR. Recent research shows the most empirical evidence for the working-memory hypothesis. The theory posits that retrieving a memory of an event requires limited-capacity working memory resources. If a secondary task is executed during a retrieval that shares this dependence, fewer resources will be available for recalling the memory, and the latter will be experienced as less vivid and emotional (van den Hout et al., 2011). The eye movements and the recall of a traumatic memory are concurrent; this dual task reduces the vividness and emotionality of the traumatic image (van den Hout & Engelhard, 2011; Gunter & Bodner, 2008).

In administering the EMDR protocol, the therapist asks focused questions designed to activate memories of the trauma. Distractive bilateral stimulation (e.g., eye movements, hand taps) is then used to evoke more appropriately functional trauma-related associations, thus helping to neutralize the traumatic memories.

The EMDR procedure is protocol driven. In the assessment phase, the therapist helps clients to choose the most distressing image of the traumatic history. Together they identify the *negative cognition* that the clients still generate about themselves while viewing that mental image. A picture is drawn of the most distressing mental image. The clients are asked what *positive cognition* they would prefer to have instead, and how valid or believable that cognition is. Then the client is asked what emotion is triggered when looking at the mental image with the negative cognition in mind, where he can feel it in his body and how distressing the image is on a scale from 0 to 10. The desensitization phase can now begin, using the external stimuli. The clients are asked to report the sensations this procedure evokes (e.g., images, sounds, emotions). This sets the healing process sufficiently in motion to enable information processing. During this desensitization phase, the therapist also assesses how much tension the original image still provokes working with scale from 0 to 10. If the memory has been neutralized, the positive cognition is then "installed" by focusing on this cognition and the client is asked for more positive associations. A "body scan" is then made to determine whether the client is still experiencing tension. The EMDR session then ends (ten Broeke & de Jongh, 1999).

DEAFNESS AND MENTAL HEALTH
PROBLEMS OF DEAF CLIENTS

The number of deaf and severely hard of hearing people in the Netherlands has been estimated at 11,400 in a population of about 16 million (de Graaf, Knippers &

Bijl, 1997). Sign language has developed greatly in recent years (Koenen et al., 1998). Deaf children in the Netherlands are now addressed bilingually (in Dutch Sign Language and spoken Dutch) in order to make sign language accessible to them and lay the groundwork for learning spoken and written Dutch. Many deaf children use a cochlear implant (CI) these days, giving rise to many new choices, possibilities, and cultural and psychological challenges (Blume, 2006; Tijsseling, 2006). In addition, parents with a strong sense of self-worth are having a positive effect on the social competence of their deaf children (Hintermair, 2013). However, the responsibility of making early choices in creating a signing environment for their deaf children, the parents' grieving process, and the decision to opt for a CI operation all detract from parents' feelings of competence. Many deaf people report that the development of their attachment to their parents was more complex than that of hearing children. It is not yet clear whether this derives from the role of sound in early attachment or from the social exclusion that results from not being able to hear or from both. Because deafness has so much impact on all family members and their relationships with one another, a systemic approach is essential to any therapeutic interaction with deaf people.

Deaf culture (Kyle, 1990; Padden & Humphries, 2005) gives the deaf population a social context and imparts healing qualities as a place where one is neither different nor excluded. Tijsseling (2006) points out that deaf people do not automatically join this community; they all decide for themselves. In the course of a deaf individual's life, the individual will at times feel more need or less need to be part of the deaf community.

On the whole, deaf and hard of hearing people are two to four times more susceptible to mental illness than hearing people (Fellinger, Holzinger, & Pollard, 2012; de Graaf, Knippers, & Bijl, 1997; van Eldik, 1998; van Gent et al., 2007). Because they cannot hear, they do not acquire and employ language or social conventions as readily as hearing people. Despite the fact that sign language affords deaf people access to language and culture, the gap between deaf and hearing people is still wide due to the predominance of spoken language, ignorance, and prejudice. Since deaf people feel excluded from many social groups, including their own wider families, and are often insecure about interacting with hearing people, many may experience trauma from social impairment in addition to "ordinary" traumas. Also, being deprived of information about an event can be traumatizing. A useful concept for clients in such cases is *information deprivation trauma* (Schild & Dalenberg, 2012). In the Netherlands, deaf clients have access to numerous supportive services to deal with social or medical issues, but these resources do not necessarily address trauma issues.

Common psychiatric diagnoses in deaf people are depression, anxiety, PTSD, and adjustment and personality disorders (de Bruin & de Graaf, 2004). Prevalence rates of psychiatric cases (49%) and *DSM-IV* disorders (27% emotional, 11% behavioral, and 7% other conditions) have been found in deaf children (van Gent et al., 2007). In addition, deaf subjects demonstrate more symptoms of depression and anxiety than hearing subjects (Kvam, Loeb, & Tambs (2006).

Because people with early onset deafness may experience a very different process of cognitive, social, and linguistic development, it is not always easy to make "pure" diagnoses, especially in personality disturbances. Another important point is that an Axis II diagnosis may lead to discrimination or stigmatization of deaf people, although such was not intended by the authors of the *Diagnostic and Statistical Manual of Mental Disorders (DSM)*.

During the treatment process, many deaf clients report difficulties with raising their hearing children. The "hearingness" of their children can give rise to complex hierarchical conflicts. For deaf parents, as well as their hearing children, confused feelings about responsibility, sense of belonging, identity, and loyalty issues may result (Preston, 2000; Schultz Myers, Myers, & Marcus, 1999). The hearing child of deaf parents might also benefit greatly from a therapist with knowledge of deafness and deaf culture since the hearing child of deaf parents "feels deaf inside and hearing outside."

THERAPEUTIC ASPECTS OF WORKING WITH DEAF CLIENTS

In any therapy, ease of communication between therapist and client is essential. For deaf and hard of hearing clients, the therapist should have a command of several different communication resources (in our case Dutch Sign Language and Sign-Supported Dutch), as well as clear articulation and a clear speech communication attitude (i.e., looking deaf clients straight in the eye, avoiding backlighting, using shorter sentences). It is also important that a hearing therapist have an open, cross-cultural attitude. Since this is a minority culture, sensitivities exist that could be detrimental to the therapeutic relationship and undermine the effectiveness of the treatment. Common impediments are a "hearing-knows-best" attitude, denial of the psychological damage caused by hearing people, linguistic misinterpretations, and a failure to notice when a client does not understand. In other words, professionals who work with deaf people need to adopt a culturally affirmative approach (Glickman & Gulati, 2003).

ADAPTING CONVENTIONAL TECHNIQUES

Several considerations are important in adapting conventional therapeutic techniques to the deaf client group:

- Many interventions are highly language based, including behavioral analyses, journal forms, written assignments, and psychological test materials. Deaf clients often have problems with written Dutch since sign language has a very different grammatical structure. For writing assignments or journal forms, deaf clients may be allowed to use their own sign language grammar. Therapists can also suggest that their deaf clients videotape their assignments. This may help them do the assignments in a sufficiently relaxed manner to make these suitable for use in language-based interventions.

- Questionnaires and tests can be translated into sign language. One problem here is the relatively small size and heterogeneous nature of the client group (in terms of types of deafness, language use, and cultural orientation). Another difficulty is the lack of validated standards. Moreover, the sign language style of the person administering a questionnaire can influence a client's answering behavior (Brauer, 1992). Brauer has reported that an exuberant signer obtained lower depression scores than a modest signer when administering the Minnesota Multiphasic Personality Inventory (MMPI) to statistically comparable groups of clients.

- If an assignment to be done as part of the therapy is unclear, visual or physical examples may be used to clarify it. The influence of negative thoughts, for example, may be clarified by using a physical exercise; a family problem becomes more tangible through the use of small figurines representing the family members; a picture drawn on a board can speak volumes.

- Another visually oriented technique is to make a video recording and then play it back and discuss it. This can help deaf clients correct certain behaviors in non-threatening ways, thereby alleviating their symptoms.

PTSD IN DEAF CLIENTS

Deaf participants in a study (Schild & Dalenberg, 2012) had a high rate of unique trauma-type experiences (average 6.18, SD = 2.65). Higher levels of trauma exposure were associated with more depression, anger, irritability, sexual concerns, tension-reduction behaviors, and substance-abuse problems. In a retrospective Norwegian study (Kvam, 2004), deaf females aged 18–65 who lost their hearing before the age of 9 ($N = 177$) reported sexual abuse with contact before the age of 18 more than twice as often as hearing females, and deaf males more than three times as often as hearing males. The abuse of the deaf children was also more serious. Very few cases were reported to parents, teachers, or authorities.

Although traumatic experiences are rated as high, Schild and Dalenberg (2012) found that only 19.5% of their sample met the PTSD diagnostic criteria (compared to 25–30% in traumatized hearing individuals). They found only avoidance/numbing and hyperarousal symptoms to predict the presence of PTSD; reexperiencing symptoms did not. Thus PTSD appears to manifest itself differently or in a different symptom constellation among deaf individuals, possibly because they are experiencing more chronic (as opposed to acute) symptoms. Also, certain

PTSD criteria (e.g., reactivity to internal and external cues and feelings of detachment) might not be predictive within the deaf population since these are more common experiences.

Interestingly, the subjects in this study (ibid.) also reported significantly more symptoms of dissociation. No significant differences occurred between low- and high-trauma groups, and no significant correlation existed between the amount of trauma experienced and dissociation. Dissociation is apparently used as a defense mechanism in coping with highly emotional experiences. This might partly be due to the deaf population's expectation of having little influence on their environment and the difficulties they experience in forming psychological concepts due to information deprivation (Rieffe et al., 2009).

In diagnosing and treating PTSD in deaf clients it seems crucial to be aware of the risk of under- or misdiagnosing and to be attentive to the specific presentation of traumatic experiences and PTSD symptoms. This stresses the importance of the clinical interview by a sufficiently signing clinician.

EMDR FOR DEAF CLIENTS

EMDR treatment focuses on the images and memories in a client's mind and body. This means that clients must be able to express themselves in their own language and image level during the EMDR without having to adapt to someone else's language. This is a great boon to deaf clients, given the large amount of adaptation that is generally expected of them. Obviously this also requires that the therapist be highly proficient in sign language in order to follow what a client is saying.

The instructions given while administering the EMDR protocol are repetitive. Clients quickly learn what is expected of them. Again, little emphasis is put on language use, which has the advantage of avoiding confusion and distraction.

Using the EMDR protocol in sign language involves a number of linguistic challenges. During the desensitization phase, for example, the question "What comes up?" is asked. In sign language, however, one cannot ask that unspecific question without localizing the gesture somewhere. Making the sign near your head refers to thoughts or ideas, near your heart refers to emotions, and near your stomach implies physical experiences. This makes the question less open than is intended in the protocol; the client must have the opportunity to follow where "the pain" is localized. One solution is to make all three gestures. On the other hand, making the sign at a certain location may also be a subtle way of investigating other loci of experience, as in situations where a client "gets stuck."

Another significant difficulty is that the search for negative cognitions requires more explanation to deaf clients than to hearing ones. Some deaf people grow up in impoverished language environments where using abstractions and rising above one's own experience are not daily fare. One risk of this partly linguistic impairment is that the therapist may excessively influence the content of what the deaf client identifies as negative and positive cognitions. That would deprive the client of the chance to articulate accurate, personally meaningful cognitions. Hearing therapists can benefit from consulting native signers about how best to express certain negative and positive cognitions in sign language. A distressing fact at a more general level is that many deaf clients have considerable difficulty expressing positive views of themselves at all. This can clearly come to light in EMDR because the protocol explicitly requires such cognitions. This problem underlines how strongly people with hearing impairments are brought up to adapt to the hearing world and how little specified positive feedback they receive about their own functioning. This is also an important lesson for other types of therapy, as well as for child rearers, who can translate it into affirmative action with regard to their children.

As to the bilateral stimulation technique, obviously it is not possible to use auditory stimuli. The therapist must have recourse to eye movements and tactile stimuli. During the sometimes heavily emotional desensitization phase, hearing clients can be stimulated to push ahead by the use of certain sounds or spoken encouragement. This is less straightforward with deaf clients. Since they need their eyes to follow the therapist's fingers, any other signs or gestures made now might break their concentration and trigger a new conversation. To get deaf clients to persevere and move ahead with the desensitization, the therapist can make encouraging nods, lightly touch their elbow, or raise the thumb of the other hand.

Our experiences with EMDR so far indicate that deaf clients may process and store traumatic events differently from hearing clients. They seem to store them more as physical material. As a result, some deaf people will reexperience the trauma during EMDR in mainly physical ways. Ferocious physical reactions may ensue; they may tremble violently and experience anew the motions and physical sensations that accompanied the trauma. Abreaction or reenactment may occur. Consider this example: During an EMDR session with a female deaf client who had been traumatized by being locked up in a cellar, the client began banging her fists on the consulting room door and crawling in misery across the floor. Such episodes require robustness on the part of the therapist and clear agreements about the limits of physical contact with the therapist ("It's fine to hold my hand if things get difficult, but you're not allowed to hurt me").

THE THERAPY

In the following case example, I highlight some of the specific psychological consequences that deafness can have, and I demonstrate how traumatized deaf clients can benefit from EMDR. I also argue that a systemic, family approach is indispensable in treating this client group.

~

MOTHER (SALISA)

Salisa is a congenitally deaf Afro-Amerind Surinamese woman living in the Netherlands. At age 27, she requested assistance from us with problems in bringing up her 9-year-old hearing daughter, Chanti. With a history of heart disease since birth, Chanti had been operated on 6 months earlier. The operation was successful, but Chanti was left with a large scar on her chest. Since the operation, she had been having concentration problems at school, was afraid to sleep by herself, was impudent to her mother, was agonizing about why heart disease had to happen to her, and suffered from extreme needle phobia. She was bullied at school because she was embarrassed to undress for PE.

Salisa was very troubled about her daughter and felt unable to cope with Chanti's nighttime fears, her problems at school, and refusing to listen to her. She also reported that she herself panicked whenever Chanti got sick or even seemed to be coming down with a minor ailment. Salisa also has a 4-year old son, Chris, whose father, though remaining involved, was not living with the family.

Salisa was born deaf because her mother (M) had rubella during pregnancy. Salisa had spent the early years of her life in Surinam and had attended deaf school there. Both M and the school were strongly focused on adapting to the hearing world and mastering spoken Dutch. Signing was discouraged at school under threat of physical punishment, but the deaf schoolmates still used it in secret. As a result, Salisa was now fluent in sign language, but she used her voice whenever hearing people were around.

Salisa had felt very much at home with the other children in the deaf schools in Surinam and the Netherlands. She also felt close to her deaf cousin, more so than to her own sister. But she had no other deaf friends. She strongly looked up to hearing people and did her best to be as "hearing" as possible. In her view, having deaf friends or a deaf partner would have just made her more deaf. And when she would get tired of always adjusting, she still had her deaf cousin to fall back on. She could then express herself in sign language.

Salisa's mother, M, had decided to move to the Netherlands with her two daughters because, after a certain point, the deaf school in Surinam had little more to offer. One consequence was that Salisa's father, who was peripheral to the family in any case, was now no longer in the picture at all. Nonetheless, M did her utmost to support her deaf daughter in all of her life tasks. In cases where her daughter was unable to make decisions because of her lack of information, M took over. This pattern continued even after Salisa reached adulthood. This sometimes aroused resentment in her younger, hearing sister.

Salisa met Chanti's father when she was 17. Neither Salisa nor the boyfriend's parents were happy with their children's choice of partner. His parents objected to the fact that Salisa was deaf and also had a different religion. M was angry because her daughter was being rejected by the boyfriend's parents. When Salisa unexpectedly became pregnant with Chanti, the relationship with the boyfriend's parents came under great pressure. The parents wanted Salisa to get an abortion, and that infuriated both Salisa and her family.

The relationship did not last. Salisa's attempts to build her own life with Chanti's father soon failed because of the family animosities. Once again M took control. Soon after, Chanti was born and was diagnosed with congenital heart problems. Salisa is still very upset by the fact that Chanti's father shunned all involvement with his daughter's birth and illness.

∾

CHANTI (THE HEARING DAUGHTER)

Chanti was happy that she could communicate with her mother so well. While shopping, she helped her if Salisa had trouble understanding the salespeople. If there was a parent interview at school, Chanti went along to translate. Everyone was impressed that she did this so well. But Chanti did not like it when relatives told her to take good care of her mother. At night she felt scared because her bedroom was downstairs and her mother's upstairs. If anything were to happen, then her mother would not hear her calls for help. After the operation, Chanti refused to sleep alone downstairs anymore. Chanti was also very strict with her little brother, Chris. When her mother allowed him to go outside with Chanti to play, Chanti spoke harshly to him if he did not obey her. At home, her mother did not approve of Chanti's sharp words. Chanti appeared confused as to when she could boss Chris about and when not.

Salisa had a strong desire to be a good mother. She dressed her children impeccably and tried to instill in them the highest values and norms. At the time she and Chanti were living with M, Salisa had a lot of trouble accepting M's interference in Chanti's upbringing. Because M could understand Chanti's spoken language and Salisa could not, Salisa tended to feel inferior. She wanted to prove she could bring up Chanti just as well as M. The wider family also kept a sharp eye on Salisa's ability to cope with the childrearing.

∾

DSM DIAGNOSES OF SALISA AND CHANTI

We diagnosed Salisa with an Axis I parent-child relational problem and with PTSD. We postponed Axis II diagnosis in view of her dependent relationship with her mother; avoidant behavior might be seen to some degree as part of the deaf cultural context. On Axis III we noted her deafness, and on Axis IV her problems in the primary support group and her occupational problems. Chanti was diagnosed with Axis I parent-child relational problems and a specific phobia. On Axis III we described her heart problems.

TREATMENT PROCESS

After presentation, Salisa was assigned to a deaf therapist. Her mother accompanied her to the first session. After seeing that the therapist could communicate well with her daughter, she departed with a sense of relief. Although Salisa felt gratified that the deaf therapist could communicate well, she seemed to have trouble believing that a deaf person could also be an expert. When a sign language–competent hearing therapist joined the sessions for the family interviews and the EMDR, Salisa immediately adapted her behavior by refraining from signing and by using voice communication only. At that point the deaf therapist could no longer understand what Salisa was saying. The deaf therapist repeatedly took an assertive stance during the family interviews whenever she could no longer follow the conversation. In so doing, she demonstrated to Salisa behavioral alternatives for interacting with hearing people. Later in the therapy, we would address Salisa's self-esteem as a deaf person.

Before the EMDR sessions for both Salisa and her daughter, Salisa was asked to write down both of their trauma histories. But since she did not feel sufficiently secure in writing Dutch, she instead told (in sign language) both histories to the deaf therapist, who then recorded them in written Dutch. This allowed Salisa to take a first step in working through the trauma in her own language and within a deaf cultural context and without feeling rejected by the hearing therapist who was later to administer the EMDR.

One critical problem now facing Salisa's family was that Chanti was highly fearful of an approaching hospital appointment where blood was to be drawn. This kept Chanti awake at night, and Salisa was dreading the appointment, too. They had already postponed the appointment several times. As a consequence of her congenital heart disease, Chanti already had plenty of experience with both injections and blood tests. She had never liked getting shots, but her fear of blood tests dated from the day when a medical student could not find her vein and had to poke her arm several times. Although the student finally succeeded, the process was very painful.

Given the heavy tension in the family caused by the upcoming lab appointment, we decided to address Chanti's needle phobia first. We hypothesized that Salisa's stress would ease once her daughter became less anxious and began sleeping better.

Chanti's EMDR

As her most distressing mental image of the trauma, Chanti chose the moment when the painful needle was inside her arm and the blood was flowing into the test tube. With some effort, we articulated "I am powerless" as a negative cognition and "I can handle it" as a positive cognition. We decided on hand taps for the bilateral stimulation. Chanti had few associations in between hand taps but could always articulate well which aspect of the distressing image provoked tension: how the needle makes a bump in her skin, how much it hurts, how the blood flows into the test tube. In the course of the EMDR process, Chanti cheered up and had fun doing the hand taps. By the end of the session, she was proud she had learned to process the distressing image—that she had succeeded in doing something that difficult. She then felt up to the necessary trip to the hospital.

Following the session, though, we learned that the family was still not keeping the appointment for the blood test. It turned out that Salisa was still dreading the hospital visit and that we had been wrong in our hypothesis that her stress was linked to that of her daughter. Delving further, we discovered that going to the hospital evoked in her a formidable array of distressing images. These stemmed from the horrific year she had gone through after Chanti was born with heart problems and after Chanti's father had let her down. Together we searched for the most disturbing images from that period of her life.

With the deaf therapist, she formulated two trauma stories, one about her daughter's history of illness and one involving the breakup with her partner. The first story brought to light her desperate attempts to get across to the doctors that something was wrong with her baby. They did not take her seriously due to the difficult communication involving her deafness. She had to go back and implore them several times to examine Chanti before they finally admitted Chanti to the hospital and diagnosed her with severe heart disease. The image of the first time she saw her baby connected to a battery of monitors was still etched in Salisa's memory. She feared for her baby's life. In retrospect, it was clearly her own tenacity that saved Chanti's life. This made Salisa feel both angry and proud.

Salisa's First EMDR

The first EMDR session with Salisa addressed Chanti's history of illness. It was agreed beforehand that any images and emotions that might surface involving her ex-partner would be postponed until a following EMDR session. The most distressing image was that of Chanti in the hospital bed—an image with a high affective valence for Salisa. During the therapy she at first found it difficult to express her negative cognition of herself. Her main focus was "My child is in danger." When we searched further for her cognition of herself, we discovered that she felt terribly powerless. During the EMDR process, the many tears that she had not cried at the time of Chanti's illness came to the surface, and so did her anger toward the doctors who did not take her seriously, as well as the excruciating fear of losing her daughter. Although we did touch on her feeling of standing there all alone, without Chanti's father, we did not work through that emotion just yet. Although Salisa's memory of Chanti in the hospital bed was to remain a distressing image after the EMDR, she did succeed in removing the charge from the emotions surrounding it.

Salisa felt very relieved after the EMDR treatment. She noticed that she no longer reacted so tensely when Chanti developed brief ailments. She was also able to cope more calmly with Chanti's problems at school and help her deal with them. Ultimately she also managed to keep the hospital appointment. Both she and Chanti still found it slightly scary, but they were proud of themselves when they managed to get through it with no real problems. Even the blood test went well.

Once the hospital problems were solved, it came out that Chanti was jealous of her brother. He had a father who was active in the family, and she did not. She was also preoccupied by many questions about her own father: why did he not come to visit anymore, why had things gone wrong between her parents, who actually was her father? Questions like these upset Salisa. She could not answer them, and she was not sure whether it would be good for Chanti to know more about her father. That angered and frustrated Chanti. Salisa reported that she herself still harbored considerable rage against Chanti's father and was at a loss to deal with her daughter's anger at her. This served as an appropriate prelude to the EMDR session about her ex-partner.

Salisa's Second EMDR

The most distressing image in Salisa's narrative about her ex-partner was the scene in which he told her he wanted nothing to do with her and Chanti. The negative cognition of herself that she identified in this image was "I am nothing." During the EMDR session, a tremendous amount of anger came to the surface, and she began to feel again how humiliated she had felt by her ex and his family. Later it would also become clear how much she regretted that they were unable to take care of Chanti together, how upset she was that Chanti had no contact with him, and what she had liked so much about him. Ultimately she succeeded in experiencing the positive cognition "I'm fine the way I am" (expressed in sign language).

After this session, Salisa was able to tell Chanti more about her father. The EMDR had helped her remember what she had valued about him, and she could now convey this recollection to her daughter. Though it was difficult for her, she and her daughter began thinking together about how Chanti could seek contact with her father and his family. This gave a very positive impulse to the mother-daughter relationship. Chanti became more relaxed now that she had answers to her questions about her father.

Although she still felt sad that he was not involved in her life, she was less upset since she had been able to talk to her mother about the fact. A positive spin-off of Salisa's coming to terms with her difficult relationship with her ex was that she could now create more room for her current partner, Chris's father. That allowed him to become more involved with the family; he even moved in with them. This gave more depth to the father role in the family, and, in a modest way, he could even fulfill that role for Chanti, too.

TREATMENT RESULTS

Both the deaf mother and the hearing daughter experienced alleviation of their psychological symptoms. In this treatment we embedded the EMDR technique in a broader psychotherapeutic approach focused on the systemic context of this family. The advantage of this combined treatment is that we were able to address a broad range of symptoms within a bicultural context. We also took advantage of the child's therapeutic progress to promote further treatment of the deaf mother's PTSD symptoms. In an individual treatment her PTSD symptoms would probably not have surfaced and would therefore have remained untreated. This correlates with the research results of Schild and Dalenberg (2012), who found more avoidant/numbing reactions in deaf participants with high-trauma experiences.

The cooperation between the hearing and the deaf therapist is noteworthy since it had such positive therapeutic effects. The deaf therapist was a wonderful role model and facilitated the building of trust with the hearing therapist.

CONCLUSION

Once adapted to deaf clients linguistic and cultural context, eye movement desensitization and reprocessing (EMDR) technique can be effective in treating them, given its compatibility with the distinctive ways of storing and processing critical events used by these clients.

As illustrated in the earlier case study, communication and social interpretation skill issues, with related family relationship problems, are quick to surface in therapy with deaf clients. Learning the necessary social skills to function in a hearing society can be especially complex and confusing in families with deaf children, deaf parents, or both; thus it is virtually impossible to view deaf clients outside their familial contexts or minimize their strong impact on hearing siblings, parents, and even grandparents.

A systemic approach can accommodate the sensitivities and entanglements that exist in these contexts and provide opportunities to repair skewed relationships between deaf and hearing members of a family. This chapter illustrates how EMDR, as a therapeutic technique, can effectively contribute to this process.

REFERENCES

Blume, S. S. (2006). *Grenzen aan genezen*. Amsterdam: Uitgeverij Bakker.

Brauer, B. A. (1992). The signer effect on MMPI performance of deaf respondents. *Journal of Personality Assessment, 58*(2), 380–388.

de Bruin, E., & de Graaf, R.. (2004). What do we know about deaf clients after thirteen years of ambulatory mental health care? An analysis of the PsyDoN database, 1987–1999. *American Annals of the Deaf, 5,* 384–393.

de Graaf, R., Knippers, E. W. A., & Bijl, R. (1997). *Doofheid en ernstige slechthorendheid in Nederland: Mate van voorkomen en relevante achtergrondkenmerken* [Prevalence and relevant background characteristics of deafness and severe hardness of hearing in the Netherlands]. Utrecht: Trimbos Institute.

Fellinger, J., Holzinger, D., & Pollard, R. (2012). Mental health of deaf people. *Lancet, 379,* 1037–1044.

Glickman, N. S., & Gulati, S. (2003). *Mental health care of deaf people: A culturally affirmative approach.* Mahwah, NJ: Erlbaum.

Gunter, R. W., & Bodner, G. E. (2008). How eye movements affect unpleasant memories: Support for a working-memory account. *Behaviour Research and Therapy, 46,* 913–931.

Hintermair, M. (2013, March). *Working with families of deaf and hard of hearing children: What we know from research and practice about parents' and children's needs.* Keynote lecture at the symposium "Normal or Special?," Amsterdam.

Hout, M. A. van den, & Engelhard, I. M. (2011, April). Hoe het komt dat EMDR werkt. *Directieve Therapie, 31*(1), 5–23.

Hout, M. A. van den, Engelhard, I. M., Betsma, D., Slofstra, C., Hornsveld, H., Houtveen, J., et al. (2011, December). EMDR and mindfulness: Eye movements and attentional breathing tax working memory and reduce vividness and emotionality of aversive ideation. *Journal of Behavior Therapy and Experimental Psychiatry, 42*(4), 423–431. doi:10.1016/j.jbtep.2011.03.004

Koenen, L., Bloem, T., Janssen, R., & van de Ven, A. (Eds.). (1998). *Gebarentaal: De taal van doven in Nederland.* Amsterdam: Uitgeverij Atlas.

Kvam, M. H. (2004). Sexual abuse of deaf children: A retrospective analysis of the prevalence and characteristics of childhood sexual abuse among deaf adults in Norway. *Child Abuse & Neglect, 28,* 241–251.

Kvam, M. H., Loeb, M., & Tambs, K. (2006). Mental health in deaf adults: Symptoms of anxiety and depression among hearing and deaf individuals. *Deaf Studies and Deaf Education, 12*(1), 1–7.

Kyle, J. (1990). The deaf community: Culture, custom and tradition. In S. Prillwitz & T. Vollhaber (Eds.), *Sign language research and application* (pp. 175–186). Hamburg: Signum Press.

Padden, C. A., & Humphries, L. A. (2005). *Inside deaf culture.* Cambridge, MA: Harvard University Press.

Preston, P. (2000). *Mother father deaf: Living between sound and silence.* Cambridge, MA: Harvard University Press.

Rieffe, C., Kouwenberg, M., Scheper, I., Smit, C., & Wiefferink, K. (2009). Inzicht in de eigen emoties bij dove kinderen. *Van horen zeggen, 50,* 10–14.

Schild, S., & Dalenberg, C. J. (2012). Trauma exposure and traumatic symptoms in deaf adults. *Psychological Trauma: Theory, Research, Practice, and Policy, 4*(1), 117–127.

Schultz Myers, S., Myers, R. R., & Marcus, A. L. (1999). Hearing children of deaf parents: Issues and interventions within a bicultural context. In I. W. Leigh (Ed.), *Psychotherapy for the deaf* (pp. 121–148). Washington, DC: Gallaudet University Press.

Shapiro, F. (1989). Efficacy of the eye movement desensitization procedure in the treatment of traumatic memories. *Journal of Traumatic Stress, 2,* 199–223.

Shapiro, F. (2001). *Eye movement desensitization and reprocessing: Basic principles, protocols and procedures.* New York: Guilford Press.

ten Broeke, E., & Jongh, A. de. (1999). Eye movement desensitization and reprocessing bij posttraumatische stress-stoornissen (EMDR in PTSD). In P. G. H. Aarts & W. D. Visser (Eds.), *Trauma: Diagnostiek en behandeling* [Trauma: Diagnostics and treatment] (pp. 321–338). Houten, the Netherlands: Bohn Stafleu Van Loghum.

Tijsseling, C. (2006). *Anders doof zijn: Een nieuw perspectief op dove kinderen* [Being deaf differently: A new perspective on deaf children]. Twello, the Netherlands: Van Tricht.

van der Kolk, B. A. (1996). The body keeps the score: Approaches to the psychobiology of posttraumatic stress disorder. In B. A. van der Kolk, A. C. McFarlane, & L. Weisaeth (Eds.) *Traumatic stress: The effects of overwhelming experience on mind, body and society* (pp. 214–241. New York: Guilford Press.

van Eldik, T. (1998). *Psychische problemen, gezinsbelasting, gezinsfunctioneren en meegemaakte stress bij dove kinderen* [Mental health problems, family stress, family functioning and stressful life events of deaf children]. Voorburg/Zoetermeer, the Netherlands: Instituut voor Doven Effatha.

van Gent, T., Goedhart, A. W., Hindley, P. A., & Treffers, P. D. A. (2007). Prevalence and correlates of psychopathology in a sample of deaf adolescents. *Journal of Child Psychology & Psychiatry, 48,* 950–958.

5

Silent Wisdom: Equine-Assisted Counseling with Deaf Clients

Karen A. Tinsley

What is equine-assisted counseling (EAC)? Imagine arriving at a small country farm nestled into a hillside, surrounded by old oak trees standing sentinel over younger maples and pines. In the distance, four horses graze peacefully, while two in a nearby pasture pick up their heads to assess the new arrival. Once they determine you represent no threat, they drop their heads and continue to graze. You are greeted by a friendly dog, wiggling his way over to you for a cursory sniff. He suddenly trots off toward a person walking out of the barn in dusty jeans, waving a friendly hello. This is your counselor, and it is your first EAC session.

For the past two hundred years, horseback riding has been used as a therapeutic intervention for rehabilitating persons with physical disabilities. This approach to physical rehabilitation began appearing in the United States in the 1960s, and soon after, programs offering therapeutic riding to individuals with disabilities as a means of improving psychomotor functioning also reported improvements in socioemotional functioning (Frewin & Gardiner, 2005). This recognition has led to a recent growth in the industry which offers opportunities for human-equine interaction in which the human feet remain on the ground. The power of this approach lies in the relationship between the client and the horse. During a session that is monitored closely by the therapeutic team, consisting of a licensed mental health clinician and an equine specialist, client and horse depend on nonverbal cues to interact effectively during the experiential-based therapeutic session. The licensed mental health clinician brings the psychological expertise to the session, and the equine specialist provides expertise in the behavior and handling of the horses. The team works in concert to ensure the emotional and physical safety of both human and horse as they complete an assigned "challenge" task.

As equine-assisted counseling has gained popularity, it has reached families, military personnel, youth groups, and individuals of all ages. Given the nonverbal nature of this therapeutic approach, it was assumed that Deaf clients could also benefit. In 2009 PBJ Connections, Inc., was approached by a signing clinician from the St. Vincent Family Center to refer several Deaf families for EAC sessions. Having participated in a Deaf group demonstration in Maine, the Deaf services clinician was eager to share cultural expertise with the willing nonprofit organization in Ohio. Through the use of interpreters, sessions were provided as an adjunct service to case management and therapy for two families. As a result of the positive feedback, collaboration between PBJ Connections and the Deaf Services Program led to a small grant-sponsored project for Deaf families. Upon completion of this pilot program, additional grant-sponsored collaborations occurred between PBJ Connections and the Ohio School for the Deaf and, more recently, with a local Deaf-oriented community resource.

RATIONALE

Why horses? Current literature cites the unique qualities of these prey animals as key factors in their success as partners in EAC sessions. The primary concern of any prey animal is safety. It is biologically designed to survive by *fight, flight,* or *freeze* reactions. Humans also have these abilities, but as our brains evolved and developed a more complex cerebral cortex, we also expanded our ability to use defense mechanisms such as rationalization, projection, and minimization to manage the more primal responses (Cozolino, 2010). In contrast, the prey animal's senses remain finely tuned to catch subtle nuances in the environment. These senses in turn stimulate the adrenal system into taking appropriate action. Although intelligent and sentient, the horse does not have a human's capacity for logical reasoning (McGreevy & McLean, 2010). The horse reacts *without* the influence of cognitive filtering, which gives EAC sessions their uniqueness. When the horse is allowed to express its natural instincts, clients have an opportunity to examine their own reactions and explore whether these reactions are part of a pattern of coping that may or may not be serving them well in other aspects of their lives. For example, if a client approaches a horse in a state of high energy (positive or negative), it will most likely react by moving away until it feels safe. For a child struggling with ADHD, approaching the horse may become a lesson in self-regulation as the horse reacts to the child's symptoms.

Much like a family system, the herd functions within a hierarchy of authority that is punctuated with various alliances and conflicts among its members. The fluid dynamics of the herd change according to which horses are grouped together. Additionally, each horse's personality will influence its role in the herd and whether it exhibits assertion or aggression, passivity and compliance, or frustration and annoyance. Human clients also contribute to the herd dynamics by influencing the horse's behavior during a session. With conscientious selection of horses and careful planning by the clinical team, these sessions often evolve to reflect similar patterns of interaction within the client's relationships.

For horses in the wild, stability is a means of conserving energy and resources. The social nature of the horse leads it to create or maintain a sense of emotional equilibrium for the herd. Some horses will act as "peacekeepers" by, for example, physically intervening between two potential adversaries or providing comfort to one lower in the herd (Lesté-Lassere, 2010). Horses can evidence empathy (Grandin, 2009), as in standing guard over a sleeping pasture mate, showing concern for others, or becoming depressed over the death of a herd member. Given these qualities of self-preservation and empathy, horses can model therapeutic responses to positive and negative human social interactions or behaviors. As an active participant in the sessions, the horse reacts to the emotional environment as well as to the client's physical actions. If a husband and wife become argumentative, the horse may walk between them in an attempt to "mediate" or may simply "check out" and walk away to a "safer" distance. For a group struggling to figure out how to work together to select and catch one horse out of a pair, the more curious horse may start pawing at an overlooked halter, seeming to help the group achieve its goal. Clients are able to measure their effectiveness by such immediate responses.

The premise of equine-assisted counseling programs is to use these observations and interactions as a source of metaphorical bridging of the client's emotional and cognitive state. For example, a horse may be actively contributing to a client's distraction from processing a session. Not many clients can resist reaching out to touch this gentle giant who has decided to sniff their sleeve. What are the distractions and temptations in the clients' lives that pose challenges for them? How are they choosing to handle these challenges? The clinical team may set up a metaphorical challenge for a client within the arena: Lead the horse over a low pole without a rope and halter. Observations of how the client and the horse interact in a few EAC sessions can provide rich clinical information that may have taken months to reveal in a traditional office setting (Ewing, MacDonald, Taylor, & Bowers, 2007; Kersten, 2010; Mann & Williams, 2002; Myers, 2004).

THEORETICAL APPLICATIONS

Equine-assisted counseling has its roots in experiential counseling approaches, in which individuals put themselves in situations that challenge them mentally, physically, and emotionally in order to overcome perceived obstacles and gain insight. Equine-assisted counseling is not limited to a particular counseling theory; it is the clinician's scope of training that provides the theoretical framework, which may also include other practices such as brief therapy, gestalt, reality therapy, and

Adlerian therapy (Trotter, 2012). In addition, aspects of humanistic, experiential, family systems, cognitive behavioral therapies, and psychodynamic theories have influence in this practice. Both EAGALA and PATH International assume that licensed mental health clinicians will practice in accordance with the scope of their training and license. Because of this, EAC programs are able to effectively reach a wide variety of clients.

After reviewing multiple counseling theories, Cozolino (2010) concludes that, regardless of theoretical modality, successful therapeutic intervention comprises four common factors: *empathic attunement, optimal stress, integration of affect and cognition,* and *co-construction of narratives* (see Figure 1). These factors can also be found in EAC sessions. The horse-human interaction of EAC demands a certain level of *empathic attunement* on the part of all present, which is developed by means of the relationships and interactions between the horse and the client. When a family is not communicating effectively, and a mother gets shut out of the discussion, the horse may put its head on her shoulder as if to give her a hug of support. The reactions of the other family members can provide insight into their familial relationships. When a horse calmly approaches an anxiety-ridden teenager, it may stand still to accept careful grooming. The teen's breathing slows and deepens with each rhythmic stroke, and a sense of trust begins to form between the two. When a youth who struggles with authority begins to handle a reluctant donkey aggressively, the animal may bolt away. This honest reaction gives the youth a chance to rethink his approach; he offers a soft apology to the donkey as they attempt to establish a more collaborative relationship.

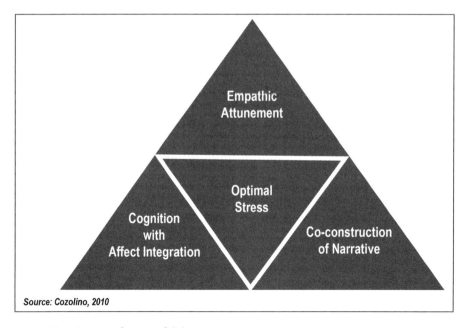

FIGURE 1.   Factors of successful therapeutic interventions.

The planned activities or "challenge" tasks of the EAC session provide an opportunity to experience controlled periods of *optimal stress.* This is when the neurobiological environment of the brain is most receptive to growth and change (Cozolino, 2010). For example, a single parent, not comfortable in her role, is given an opportunity to practice giving directives to her child through a collaborative activity that moves a horse through an obstacle course. A youth with low self-esteem is given an opportunity to have a horse follow him willingly without the use of any lead rope or treats. A group of teenagers is given an opportunity to work together to round up several wayward donkeys and bring them into an arena. These challenge tasks are designed to nudge the clients into a moderate zone of discomfort, where they are then motivated to find an emotional equilibrium and develop new insights as they attempt to reach their goal for the session. The clinical team monitors and, if necessary, modifies the sessions in order to maintain *optimal* levels of stress for both the client and the horse.

In the EAC session, clients have an opportunity to *integrate affect and cognition* as they experience events with the clinical team. The challenge tasks provide opportunities for the observation of behaviors, emotions, patterns, and physical sensations, but without therapeutic guidance to identify and acknowledge these observations, the session simply becomes a recreational period. "Catharsis without cognition does not result in integration" (Cozolino, 2010, p. 47). The role of the equine specialist may be to verbalize a horse's fearful behavior in reaction to a parent who is "just fine!" in order to highlight the observed contradictions. A mental health clinician may explore a client's teary reaction to a horse walking away from her, perhaps struggling with issues of rejection in her own life. A group of youths may become frustrated with repeated "failure" when a horse keeps knocking a pole off its standards when stepping over it. Interacting with the horse often heightens emotion in clients, helping clinicians reach those who may have been less engaged or even blocked in their treatment while in traditional therapeutic settings (see Figure 2).

The fourth factor, *co-construction of narratives,* occurs on two levels. The first takes place in the immediate session, as the client interacts with the horse: exploring, processing, and ultimately integrating her thoughts and feelings to come to some inner conclusion about the horse, about the interactions, about herself. The second level develops over the course of several sessions, as the interactions modulate and evolve to a point where the client is able to generalize and apply insights from EAC sessions to other aspects of her life. The narrative facilitates the integration of multiple neural networks through memory, language, and affect toward more productive means of functioning.

RESEARCH

Even though the field of equine-assisted counseling has grown in the past 20 years, research that supports its efficacy has been difficult to obtain, given the difficulties

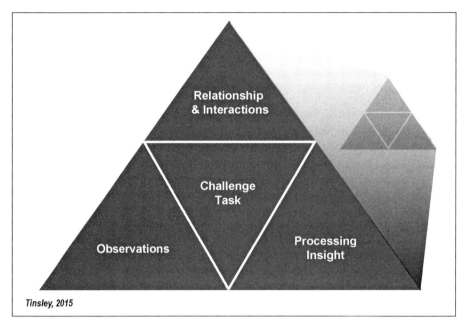

FIGURE 2.   Applications of equine-assisted counseling for successful therapeutic interventions.

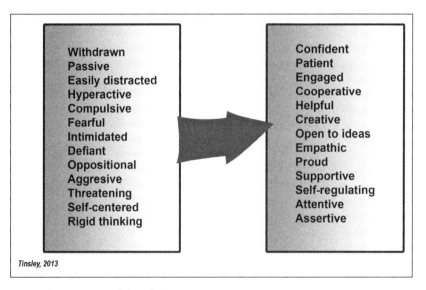

FIGURE 3.   Changes in Deaf client behaviors.

of deciding what and how to measure the pertinent human behaviors involved. Professional organizations such as EAGALA and PATH International are helping to standardize the field of equine therapy, and the International Society for Equitation Science (ISES) is encouraging scholarly equine research. Future research results may come from the contributions of social neuroscience, which describes the interconnectedness of neurology, physiology, and psychology and its impact on our social functioning. Current trauma-focused research on neural plasticity and how the brain forms new, healthier connections during therapy may provide some answers as to *why* equine-assisted counseling is so effective; however, very few EAC programs have the luxury of sufficient time, resources, and participants to obtain clinically significant data. Of the few studies that have been conducted, several stand out.

Trotter, Chandler, Goodwin-Bond, and Casey (2008)

A comparative study of 164 high-risk youth were given 12 weeks of either EAC or a classroom-based behavioral curriculum. The Behavioral Assessment Scale for Children (BASC) was used to measure pre- and postprogram changes. Results indicated that the EAC group had overall improvements in more areas of functioning, as rated by both the youths and their parents, than did the classroom-based group, which showed improvements in a few areas but were different from those of the EAC group.

Schultz, Remick-Barlow, and Robbins (2007)

A pilot study of 63 children, with and without a history of abuse or domestic violence, received an average of 19 EAC sessions. The study used the Global Assessment of Functioning (GAF) Scale and reported that improvements between pre- and post-GAFs were statistically significant and that the youngest participants and the number of sessions showed positive correlations with improved GAF scores.

Klontz, Bivens, Leinart, and Klontz (2007)

A study of 31 individuals in residential treatment received group therapy EAC sessions. Using the Brief Symptom Inventory (BSI) Severity Scale, results showed that 60% were in the clinical range prior to treatment, whereas only 20% were in the clinical range after treatment, and at a 6-month follow-up, scores rose to only 27% within clinical range.

Deaf EAC Research

In 2009 PBJ Connections and the Deaf Services Program at St. Vincent's Family Center attempted to measure pre- and postprogram outcomes for 12 participating families. Measures of adaptive and maladaptive functioning were obtained by using the Achenbach System of Empirically Based Assessment (ASEBA) forms. Despite administrative problems that compromised the data, the overall response from families was favorable. The experience highlighted a number of issues inherent in Deaf subjects (Tinsley & Jedlicka, 2012) and were revisited in 2011 by using the Behavioral Assessment Scale for Children (BASC-2), which is addressed later.

Accommodating the Deaf Client Assessments

Considerable difficulty was encountered when attempting to create a statistically sound assessment of the efficacy of EAC with Deaf clients. The ASEBA was already in use by the St. Vincent Family Center and considered a logical use of resources when it collaborated on a grant with PBJ Connections to serve 12 Deaf families. The ASL version was not available, however, and therefore required translation for many of the Deaf participants. Additionally, administration protocols were affected when the Deaf Services Program underwent personnel changes midstream. Overall, reports were favorable but lacked statistical confirmation. In a second attempt to obtain scholarly research data, PBJ Connections began utilizing the BASC-2 for all clients. In 2010 and 2011, it was administered to the first round of classes of students with cognitive disabilities (CD) from the Ohio School for the Deaf. Again, this required a translation of the written test for most of the Deaf participants, and administration protocol consistency was difficult to maintain as the reports were solicited from school personnel, family, and clients over a period of several weeks. The effort to manage, score, and interpret the tool, however, outweighed the limited information obtained, and since the tool also did not have normative data for Deaf individuals, it was abandoned in favor of anecdotal feedback and observations (Figure 4).

Year	Target Group	Partner	Sessions
2008-2009	Referred families	St. Vincent Family Center-Deaf Services	n/a
2009-2010	Referred families	St. Vincent Family Center-Deaf Services	10
2009-2010	At-risk High School students	Ohio School for the Deaf	n/a
Signing Clinician Utilized			
2010-2011	At-risk High School students	Ohio School for the Deaf	7
2010-2011	Middle School CD class *	Ohio School for the Deaf	8
2010-2011	High School CD class	Ohio School for the Deaf	8
2011-2012	Elementary CD class	Ohio School for the Deaf	17
2011-2012	Middle School CD class	Ohio School for the Deaf	19
2011-2012	Referred Adults	Community Resource	10

* CD-Cognitively Delayed or otherwise identified special needs   per Ohio School for the Deaf determination

FIGURE 4.   History of Deaf clients' equine-assisted counseling.

Interpreting

As a result of the favorable feedback on the initial pilot program in 2009, PBJ Connections initiated its first after-school, at-risk group with identified students from the Ohio School for the Deaf. Although the organization arranged to have an interpreter to facilitate communication with the nonsigning clinical team, it quickly became apparent that a cohesive session required more than just providing an interpreter. Though well intentioned, the alliances were perceived as weak in "Deaf credibility" simply as a result of their recent appearance within the Deaf community. To compound matters, the school struggled with transportation and scheduling conflicts, which fueled the already frustrated group of teenagers. As a result, this initial group suffered high dropout rates and limited progress.

In 2010 the signing clinician who had made the initial referrals in 2009 was brought on board to lead sessions. A contracted interpreter continued to facilitate communication between students and the nonsigning equine specialist. The presence (or absence) of an interpreter is an integral part of the Deaf community's experience and an opportunity for therapeutic discussion (Harvey, 1989). During an early session with the at-risk group, the signing clinician used her voice and did not sign in order to model alignment with the nonsigning equine specialist. This brought about puzzled looks from the students, and it was not until halfway through the session that one student voiced her confusion. The group then explained that they felt more comfortable with direct communication when an adult was capable of signing to them but understood and appreciated the need for an interpreter when the adult's signing skills were not sufficient. This opened the group up to more honest dialogue for the ensuing sessions.

The interpreter's skill and comfort around horses were also factors that needed to be addressed. Before the signing mental health clinician was contracted, PBJ Connections had been using a novice interpreter who had some previous connection with the agency; both the hearing clinician and the equine specialist assumed that the interpretation was accurately reflecting the conversations. With the addition of the signing clinician, who was also an RID Certified Interpreter, it became apparent that the interpretation was falling behind. In fact, the nature of the sessions—up to eight Deaf youths with varied linguistic abilities in an emotionally charged environment—required a more linguistically seasoned interpreter who also happened to be comfortable around horses. This became even more apparent later on, when the interpreter was not available, and the school administration offered the classroom teacher, who was not comfortable around horses. Even though the suggestion was turned down on the basis of conflicting roles (the teacher was in charge of that same class) and skill level (signing does not equal interpreting), safety concerns remained. No matter how linguistically skilled the interpreter is, effective interpretation cannot happen when the interpreter is internally distracted by concerns about personal safety. Instead, an opportunity opened up for the group to work together to make sure the nonsigning equine specialist was included and to discuss parallel communication difficulties the youths may have experienced in their lives. The "ideal" scenario, where both the mental health clinician and the equine specialist are skilled in American Sign Language, has yet to be formed for an EAC session.

Visual Accessibility

Eye contact was often a challenge when working with the Deaf clients (see Figure 5). The sessions took place either in a six-stall barn, in a large indoor arena, or outdoors on the farm, which had several outbuildings, round pens, and pastures. The common cultural attention-getting tactics such as stamping a foot, tapping a table, or flipping a light switch did not work well in such settings. The clinical team that was working with the Deaf clients therefore needed to remain alert and maneuver more quickly into the client's line of sight than they did for hearing clients. When working in groups, the clinical team would sometimes need to split up to cover more space and offer more opportunity for establishing eye contact. This is quite different from the situation in most hearing-oriented EAC programs, where the members of the clinical team often remain near each other and sometimes at a considerable distance from the client or group while they are engaged with the horse. The horse often presents a visual barrier to communication as well. Walking between family members or client and clinician, an average 16-hand horse is about 1,200 pounds of "in the way." How the Deaf client or family members react—*or not*—can provide rich clinical information about communication dynamics.

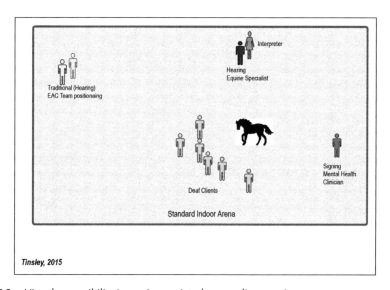

Tinsley, 2015

FIGURE 5.   Visual accessibility in equine-assisted counseling sessions.

Insight

Whereas the majority of EAC programs rely heavily on the client's ability for insight, the use of metaphors, generalization, and application of session events to the Deaf client's real-world experience have been significant challenges. Most of the Deaf clients referred to PBJ Connections were youths with behavioral and emotional issues compounded by language disfluency. Most came from homes with little or no access to sign language models, and some had cognitive impairments that impeded learning even with access to sign language. For these clients, processing had to be focused on immediate emotions and behaviors with the use of role play, modeling, and repetition. It was not unusual for the challenge task to actually commence more than halfway through the session.

MODIFICATIONS

Between 2010 and 2012 PBJ Connections collaborated with the Ohio School for the Deaf to provide group counseling sessions to specific target groups. Initially referred by the school counselor, the first two groups were a composite of at-risk high school students who had little or no interaction with each other outside the group. The following school year focused on one middle school and one high school class of students with cognitive disabilities. The plan was to develop a cohesive unit that occurred naturally as a class rather than group students with few common experiences or motivation to become cohesive. Due to the success of this design, a third year of funding provided group sessions to many of these same middle school students and a new elementary class of students with cognitive disabilities. Over time, our approach was modified and refined to meet the unique needs of each class and resulted in positive outcomes.

Structure

Although traditional EAC sessions are typically unstructured except for the assigned task, a system was extremely important to our sessions as a means of grounding students and providing a "continuity safety net" beyond which they could then explore. An opening and closing routine provided parameters for students who struggled with transitioning, attending, and predicting skills. For the elementary students, the sessions were initially segmented into "activity stations" due to the huge variations in functioning levels. Donkeys were used instead of horses because of their slower movements, smaller size, and lower reactivity. For these students, efforts were made to change only one variable per session, if at all, in order to ascertain which aspects were truly being acquired and which needed further repetition or modification.

Language

As each elementary CD student rotated to a station with adult support, the child was encouraged to develop language modeled by the adults. The target signs HAPPY, SAD, MAD, and SCARED were modeled and repeated at each station along with simple interactions. For some of the youngest participants, this was simply a chance to give an emotion a label, a sign. This pretreatment approach is known as *skills and stories* (Glickman, 2009). Although redundant to many of the adults by the third session, students who arrived with only a behavioral means of communication began to spontaneously sign in response to the interactions. By the fifth session, there were reports of spontaneous, socially appropriate *application* of these target words while at school and at home.

The middle-school CD class struggled with communicating effectively. Initial strategies were predominately incomplete phrases, directives, pointing, or physically threatening or manipulating others to their will. Socially appropriate interactions had to be modeled and encouraged. Contributing to their poor interaction skills was a remarkably poor grasp of classifiers and classifier predicates, which created misunderstandings and frustration, which in turn often led to the inappropriate behavioral expressions "typical" for this class. *How* to sign "lead the horse around the bucket" needed to be modeled for these clients. To facilitate effective communication, flash cards depicting items, horses, or people in the arena in various positions relative to each other were used to develop expressive and receptive skills as they interacted with each other. The experiential opportunities of EAC allowed these marginalized clients to feel a sense of pride as they communicated clearly to a peer, who was then able to successfully accomplish the task.

Staffing

The earlier groups were designed to have alternating sessions occur at the school. The intent was to model the successful design of the pilot family sessions from the St. Vincent Family Center, which had the support of a case manager to facilitate carryover of the session benefits. Preteaching was to be the purpose of the in-school sessions, but it became clear that students in the CD classes were struggling with the inconsistency and that disciplinary practices were too ingrained in the staff members despite efforts to keep the sessions neutral with regard to in-school issues.

For the 2011–2012 school year, all sessions were conducted at PBJ Connections. For the elementary CD class, the teacher and 1:1 education aides were encouraged to facilitate interactions with students. Initial sessions were actually used to preteach and model to *the staff* the appropriate interaction with the alingual, visually impaired, attention-challenged mix of students in their charge. The middle-school CD students, however, had a completely different set of challenges. The staff members were reluctant to remove themselves, citing behavioral histories of some of the students, when in fact it was the presence of the staff that *contributed* to the inappropriate behaviors. Once staff members were released from their monitoring duties and removed from sight, students began to explore independent problem solving without fear of being disciplined every time they made a poor choice.

~

SESSION 19: MIDDLE-SCHOOL CD CLASS

Every session began with a group meeting at a circle of cones in the arena. Over time, peer-to-peer interaction provided influential redirection for stragglers who held up the session. The selection of the horse was based on previous experience with the animal and the fact that it was smaller, slower, and more tolerant of the high-energy clients, some of whom had little awareness of their own personal-safety needs. For this session, the group was given the goal of getting the horse to walk into a 14-foot square "box" outlined on the arena floor. They were allowed to use anything in the arena, which included some long poles, cones, lunge lines, halters, lead ropes, brushes, and a few chairs, but nothing was allowed to touch the horse. This no-touch policy was put in place because of the group's tendency to rely on physical force to obtain compliance. By the time this session occurred (number 19), the "aggressive student" and the "withdrawn student" had each demonstrated emerging leadership qualities that could be capitalized on.

Although the students showed improvement working as a team, they still struggled with managing the increasing stress levels as the horse refused to walk into the "box" and thus required assistance from the clinical team to avoid group disintegration. Although a higher-functioning group might have ended without successfully completing the task, this CD group's cohesiveness was still emerging and fragile. Carryover to the next session would have cancelled out the positive experiences that were occurring in this session, as these clients would have interpreted their lingering frustration as a failure, which could have led to unwanted behaviors when they returned to school. With supportive suggestions to try something new, they were able to watch the horse calmly join them in the "box," which gave them a sense of accomplishment. This led to a group discussion about what had happened, their feelings, the contributions of each member, and why the horse might have decided to cooperate. The group then closed the session by thanking the horse and spending a few minutes patting him before selecting pieces of patterned paper to add to their horse mural. This routine-closing activity would be going back to the school on their last session as a keepsake and also served as a visual resource for continued narrative development with regard to their experiences.

∼

Adult Clients

PBJ Connections also offered limited EAC sessions to Deaf adults through a collaboration with a Deaf-oriented, nonprofit resource center. For those with uncompromised language or cognition abilities, basic scaffolding of metaphors from EAC events to life events can be a powerful experience. An energetic horse may trigger anxiety in a client, which she later realizes feels very similar to being around her abusive partner. Over several sessions, the client may discover she can take steps to ensure her safety when she is interacting with the energetic horse; she may even be able to lead it through a pattern of poles with confidence. The goal is that she be able to take that confidence, gained from being in contact with a 1,500-pound animal, and report one day that she is no longer a victim. Sometimes the outcome is not about completing a task with the horse but about communicating more effectively with a partner on how to make a situation feel safer. As a couple comes to realize that their assumptions of each other fall short of reality, they are able to develop better observation skills, leading to greater emotional attunement with each other and growth in their relationship. The use of EAC with Deaf adult clients was available for only a short funding period, but it proved worthwhile to those who participated.

CONCLUSIONS

Equine-assisted counseling can be a viable and effective mode of treatment for Deaf individuals, groups, and families. With some modifications to accommodate language, visual accessibility, and cultural sensitivity, this growing field can offer unique opportunities to a minority group that is often overlooked or swept aside in the face of clinical innovations and advances.

Future Developments

The field of EAC is evolving. With continued efforts to conduct scholarly research on its efficacy, it is gaining recognition as a feasible treatment modality. Electrocardiograms (ECGs), which measure the electromagnetic energy of the heart, have demonstrated that clients can learn not only to regulate their own levels of heart rate variability (HRV) but also influence that of others who are nearby. In a preliminary study of horse-human interaction, measurements indicated a mutual positive influence on inner state (New Meaning to "Horse Sense," 2006). With computer programs to facilitate breathing and heart-rate regulation, clients are able to master the self-regulation of their inner state and incorporate this skill in an EAC riding session, which uses music and the horse's rhythmic cadence to affect multiple neural networks simultaneously (Natural Lifemanship, 2013).

For thousands of years, horses have been "broken" through a variety of methods, many of which are outright abusive. Although horse handling has become more humane over the centuries, it is still based primarily on the negative reinforcement: the use of pressure, food-based coercion, or misplaced dominance tactics (McGreevy & McLean, 2010). Even current popular approaches that have an almost cult-like following have been shown to have weakness, however. *If current horsemanship techniques encourage the inciting of fear in order to bring about acquiescence, how is that representative of what we want clients to bring to their own relationships?* In small horsemanship circles a quiet shift is occurring to a more empathic relationship that could enhance the client's experience in an EAC session. Horsemanship through *feel* is not easy, but it is eye opening. The client gains insights through ground work as well as riding. In fact, the ground work serves as a form of preteaching. The sessions are not simply about techniques or tools but also about intent, emotional resonance, and a form of unconditional positive regard. The horse offers a level of genuine connection that can break down many walls. Not only does the client benefit, but the horse finds beneficial catharsis as well: a true partnership (Musson, 2013).

The future of equine-assisted counseling is bright and exciting. With increasing scientific support and an evolution in approaches to horsemanship, clients will have an opportunity to work through issues, improve social-emotional functioning, and gain beneficial insights. It is anticipated that Deaf clients and their families will continue to benefit from this evolved approach, and future research will hopefully substantiate that.

REFERENCES

Cozolino, L. J. (2010). *The neuroscience of psychotherapy: Healing the social brain* (2nd ed.). New York: Norton.

Equine Assisted Growth and Learning Association (EAGALA). (2012). *What is the EAGALA model?* Retrieved February 27, 2012, from http://www.EAGALA.org

Ewing, C. A., MacDonald, P. M., Taylor, M., & Bowers, M. J. (2007). Equine-facilitated learning for youths with severe emotional disorders: A quantitative and qualitative study. *Child and Youth Care Forum, 36*(1), 59–72.

Frewin, K., & Gardiner, B. (2005). New age or old sage? A review of equine-assisted psychotherapy. *Australian Journal of Counseling Psychology, 6,* 13–17.

Glickman, N. (2009). *Cognitive-behavioral therapy for deaf and hard of hearing persons with language challenges.* New York: Routledge.

Grandin, T. (2009). *Animals make us human: Creating the best life for animals.* New York: Houghton Mifflin Harcourt.

Harvey, M. A. (1989). *Psychotherapy with deaf and hard of hearing persons: A systemic model.* Hillsdale, NJ: Erlbaum.

International Society for Equitation Science. (2013). Retrieved March 18, 2013, from http://www.equitationscience.com

Kersten, G. (2010). Equine-assisted authenticity. *Equine-Assisted Networker, 4*(4), 6.

Klontz, B. T., Bivens, A., Leinart, D., & Klontz, T. (2007). The effectiveness of equine-assisted experiential therapy: Results of an open clinical trial. *Society and Animals, 15,* 257–267.

Lesté-Lassere, C. (2010, October 14). Horses reconcile, support each other after conflict. Article #17102. Retrieved February 27, 2012, from http://www.thehorse.com

Mann, D. S., & Williams, D. (2002). Equine-assisted family therapy for high-risk youth: Defining a model of treatment and measuring effectiveness. Journey Home, Inc. Walsenburg, CO: Authors.

McGreevy, P., & McLean, A. (2010). *Equitation science.* Oxford, UK: Wiley-Blackwell.

Musson, K. (2013). *The bad egg? "Well she's an appy mare . . . what do you expect?"* Retrieved March 3, 2013, from http://www.theartofriding.com/site-map/articles-applying-feel/the-bad-egg-well-she-s-an-appy-mare-what-do-you-expect

Myers, L. (2004). *Using a horse to develop recovery skills.* Retrieved March 10, 2010, from http://www.stonefoxfarm.net.hickball.html

Natural Lifemanship. (2013). *Our model.* Retrieved March 1, 2013, from http://naturallifemanship.com/?page_id=24

New Meaning to "Horse Sense." (2006). *Change of Heart, 5*(1), 1, 4. Newsletter of the Institute of HeartMath. Retrieved March 17, 2013, from http://www.equusatori.com/Body/HeartMath_artcle.pdf

Professional Association of Therapeutic Horsemanship International (PATH International). (2012). Retrieved February 27, 2012, from http://www.pathintl.org

Schultz, P., Remick-Barlow, G., & Robbins, L. (2007). Equine-assisted psychotherapy: A mental health promotion/intervention modality for children who have experienced intra-family violence. *Health & Social Care in the Community, 15*(3), 265–271.

Tinsley, K. A., & Jedlicka, H. (2012). Techniques that focus on social skills and communication: Equine assisted counseling with deaf families In K. S. Trotter (Ed.), *Harnessing the power of equine assisted counseling: Adding animal assisted therapy to your practice* (pp. 165–179). New York: Routledge.

Trotter, K. S. (Ed.). (2012). *Harnessing the power of equine assisted counseling: Adding animal assisted therapy to your practice.* New York: Routledge

Trotter, K., Chandler, C., Goodwin-Bond, D., & Casey, J. (2008). A comparative study of the efficacy of group equine assisted counseling with at-risk children and adolescents. *Journal of Creativity in Mental Health, 3*(3), 254–284.

6

Cochlear Implants: Psychosocial Implications

Irene W. Leigh

Technology can influence psychosocial functioning in many ways. The telephone, the Internet, smartphones, videophones, iPads, and many other such devices are examples of how technology has changed the way people interact with each other. For example, researchers are now analyzing the way in which social connections and loneliness are affected by reliance on the Internet (Marche, 2012). These technologies have clearly been embraced by millions of individuals.

The cochlear implant is a technological development that has long been touted as having the potential to improve deaf-hearing interactions through the use of enhanced hearing where practically none has existed (Christiansen & Leigh, 2002/2005). Researchers and professionals who focus on hearing and spoken language saw the cochlear implant as a tool that would facilitate access to education and socialization in the mainstream. However, history reveals that the development of cochlear implants was not universally welcomed, nor was it uniformly seen as a means of improving socialization and psychosocial development. We now turn to a brief history of the cochlear implant as background to clarify the impetus for research on psychosocial implications and identity formation.

A BRIEF HISTORY

Medical researchers have long desired to develop ways to remedy hearing loss, seeing this as a means of integrating deaf and hard of hearing individuals into the

Author's note: Significant portions of this chapter incorporate information presented in I. W. Leigh (2009), *A lens on deaf identities* (New York: Oxford University Press), and I. W. Leigh & D. Maxwell-McCaw (2011), Cochlear implants: Implications for deaf identities, in R. Paludneviciene & I. W. Leigh (Eds.), *Cochlear implants: Evolving perspectives* (pp. 95–110). (Washington, DC: Gallaudet University Press).

mainstream of society. Ear trumpets represented an early attempt to amplify hearing; over time such instruments evolved into hearing aids. These, however, were of limited use for those who were identified as profoundly deaf. Since at least the eighteenth century, efforts to electrically stimulate the ear included attempts to activate the auditory nerve (see Niparko & Wilson [2000] for details). Ear surgeries grew more refined over time but were effective primarily for middle ear issues. Cochlear implantation represents an evolution in this process of providing remedies for those unable to benefit from hearing aids due to inner ear issues.

After the initial reports of the actual implantation of electrodes in the cochlea during the 1950s, from France and then the United States, research on the technical and beneficial aspects of cochlear implantation gained momentum (e.g., Blume, 1999; Christiansen & Leigh, 2002/2005; Niparko & Wilson, 2000). Single-channel implantation evolved into multiple-channel implantation, starting in 1984, thereby enhancing auditory capabilities (House & Berliner, 1991; Schindler, 1999). Multi-channel cochlear implants are the standard today, and the number of bilateral cochlear implantations is increasing (Christiansen & Leigh, 2011; Roan, 2009).

In 1977 France was the site of the first pediatric implantation (Blume, 1999). One of the reasons for researching the effectiveness of cochlear implants in children during the early stages of cochlear implant research was the perception that enhancing hearing during the critical period of language acquisition would facilitate spoken language development (Christiansen & Leigh, 2002/2005).

As the deaf communities in various countries, particularly France, Australia, and the United States, became aware of these early cochlear implant efforts, opposition began to grow, based on the premise that deaf people managed to live successful lives and did not need "a repair job" on their ears (see Christiansen & Leigh, 2002/2005, for a review). Though cochlear implantation for deaf adults have become increasingly acceptable with more and more deaf adults getting implanted, considerable resistance to pediatric cochlear implantation by certain deaf community factions still exists (Christiansen & Leigh, 2011), primarily with regard to concerns about social and psychological implications (Christiansen & Leigh, 2002/2005). This is based in large part on the perception of a single-minded focus on spoken language and auditory training, with presumably serious consequences such as language acquisition delays, difficulties in socialization with hearing peers, identity confusion, and lack of in-depth connections with relevant social communities. To speak to the mental health concerns highlighted by opponents of cochlear implantation, the rest of this chapter directly addresses research that explores psychosocial adjustment as well as identity for the population of children and adolescents with cochlear implants.

RESEARCH ON PSYCHOSOCIAL ADJUSTMENT

An extensive literature explores the medical aspects of cochlear implantation, the evolving technology of the cochlear implant itself, auditory training, auditory benefits, and receptive and expressive spoken language development. An expanding corpus of research on samples of children, adolescents, and young adults with cochlear implants has explored not only listening and spoken language skills and academic achievement but also psychosocial functioning. What we can garner from the research on the latter should provide some reassurance regarding how the pediatric population is adjusting to life with cochlear implants.

Parents' and Teachers' Perceptions

Hearing parents may justify their child's cochlear implantation on the multiple potential outcomes and view the process as not necessarily precluding the option of entering the Deaf community (Berg, Herb, & Hurst, 2005; Christiansen & Leigh, 2002/2005). In contrast, they may see the refusal to implant their deaf child as limiting the child's opportunity to participate in the world of their hearing families and environment; in this regard, they do not see the implant as an impediment to psychosocial health.

Several studies have focused on parents' perceptions of how their children were functioning postimplantation (e.g., Christiansen & Leigh, 2002/2005; Nicholas & Geers, 2003; Punch & Hyde, 2011a). General conclusions indicate that parents perceive their children as exhibiting an improved quality of life, greater self-esteem, confidence, and outgoing behavior compared to preimplant. Despite these positive findings, age-appropriate socialization experiences with hearing peers were not guaranteed. Various factors potentially contributing to social difficulties included variable spoken communication skills, limited access to communication in groups due to noise, difficulties in following the course of conversations, and the attitudes of hearing peers (Bat-Chava & Deignan, 2001; Bat-Chava, Martin, & Kosciw, 2005; Chmiel, Sutton, & Jenkins, 2000; Christiansen & Leigh, 2002/2005; Kluwin & Stewart, 2000; Nicholas & Geers, 2003; Punch & Hyde, 2011a).

Studies conducted in Denmark, initially with reports from the parents of 62 children with cochlear implants and later from structured interviews with the parents of 167 additional children postimplant, indicated very satisfactory perceptions of social well-being (Percy-Smith et al., 2006; Percy-Smith, Jensen, et. al., 2008). Stronger social well-being was observed for those children who were implanted prior to 18 months of age and those using spoken language compared with those implanted after 18 months of age and who used sign-supported systems or signs only. However, due to the wide range of ages from 1 to 18 years and the lack of any breakdown by age, it is not possible to determine whether the results for the older participants implanted prior to 18 months were similar to those of the younger participants also implanted prior to 18 months.

In addition, the social well-being of 164 kindergarten and school-aged children with cochlear implants and a cohort of 2,169 hearing children was also compared, using parent questionnaires (Percy-Smith, Cayé-Thomasen, et al., 2008).

No significant difference was found between the two cohorts in overall self-esteem, number of friends, confidence, independence, social being, and happiness. Interviews with 18 parents in Finland also indicate that between 1 and 5 years after implantation, children had calmed down, were showing more self-confidence as well as enjoying an expanded social life, and were judged to be as independent as their hearing peers (Huttunen & Välimaa, 2010).

Quality of life is also measured by educational and employment history (Venail, Vieu, Artieres, Mondain, & Uziel, 2010). Using a standardized questionnaire with parents, the French researchers Venail et al. investigated the educational and employment achievements of 100 deaf children who received cochlear implants prior to age 6, most of whom were educated in the mainstream. The sample was divided into four age groups: 8–11, 12–15, 16–18, and older than 18. Of the eight in the 18+ group, four had a university-level education, and the rest had vocational training. Of some concern was the observation that 42–61% of the three groups below the age of 18 had failed a grade. Although the researchers found correlations among grade failure, pre- and postimplantation communication modes, and educational support, they noted that participants ultimately achieved educational and employment levels similar to those of their hearing peers, with a focus on spoken language as a facilitating factor. The issue of psychosocial adjustment per se was not addressed. One wonders how quality of life was affected by this high rate of grade failures. Also noteworthy is the fact that the parents—rather than the children, adolescents, and adults themselves—were the focus of this study despite the fact the offspring were old enough to respond to questions.

Punch and Hyde (2011b) are cautionary in terms of parents' perspectives regarding their children's quality of life with the cochlear implant. In their study, while the majority of parents believed their implanted children were relatively happier, less frustrated, safer, and more flexibly shared both deaf and hearing identities, Punch and Hyde note that the parents were still concerned about their children's social skills and limited participation in groups, particularly with respect to possible social isolation.

Teachers have also been involved in studies rating students with cochlear implants. Dammeyer (2010) finds that teacher ratings of a measure of psychosocial well-being in his sample of 92 Danish children with cochlear implants were comparable to the ratings for the remaining sample of 235 participants with hearing loss between 6 and 19 years of age. Additionally, Dammeyer finds that, for participants with good spoken or sign language skills, psychosocial difficulties are not substantially greater than they are for hearing children. However, the prevalence of psychosocial difficulties was 3.7 times greater for the entire sample of 334 participants compared to a hearing sample, indicating that if communication is difficult or if there are additional disabilities, adjustment becomes more problematic.

Perspectives of Pediatric Cochlear-Implant Users

Although parents' perceptions provide valuable information, studies that directly observe or ask children and adolescents with cochlear implants about their psychosocial experiences can provide more nuanced data. Basically, these studies demonstrate that, despite generally positive reports from parents as indicated earlier, children with cochlear implants observed in group situations or classroom discourse with hearing peers encounter comparatively more challenges than their hearing peers in their attempts to become active group participants (Boyd, Knutson, & Dahlstrom, 2000; Knutson, Boyd, Reid, Mayne, & Fetrow, 1997; Martin, Bat-Chava, Lalwani, & Waltzman, 2011; Preisler, Tvingstedt, & Ahlström, 2005). Acoustic challenges in the guise of noisy situations and multiple conversations contribute to difficulties that may be less prominent in one-on-one situations.

As increasing numbers of children have grown up using the cochlear implant, it is now possible to include them as study participants in research projects focusing on their development. Using this population directly, various studies incorporating interviews, questionnaires, and/or psychological measures have demonstrated generally positive psychosocial adjustment. For example, the overall quality of life for 129 children 6 years postimplant who responded to questions was revealed to be comparable to the quality of life demonstrated by hearing samples (Meserole et al., 2014). A self-report study (Nicholas and Geers, 2003) including 181 children ages 8–9 with at least 4 or more years of cochlear implant use notes that these children tended to appear competent and well-adjusted in the cognitive, physical, socioemotional, school performance, and communication domains. Interestingly, younger children and those using the most updated speech processors gave themselves higher ratings, raising the question of whether these assessments would be maintained in adolescence, when young people have a greater awareness of difficulties in communicating, particularly in noisy group situations (e.g., Sheridan, 2008). Other studies confirming the tendency for younger implanted children to rate their quality of life highly include those by Warner-Czyz, Loy, Roland, Tong, and Tobey (2009) with children between 4 and 7 years of age, and Schorr, Roth, and Fox (2009), with children aged 5 to 14 years of age who use spoken language.

In an investigation of 84 children with cochlear implants divided into two groups, the first aged 8–11 and the second aged 12–16, both cohorts scored similarly to their parents in terms of quality of life (Loy, Warner-Czyz, Tong, Tobey, & Roland, 2010). However, for the older group, the parents tended to rate their children's quality of life at school higher than the adolescents themselves did. Even though the older group of cochlear implanted children did not differ significantly from their hearing peers in quality-of-life ratings, this result suggests the possibility that the complex issues of adolescence might make these youths' perceptions of their quality of life less idealistic, particularly with regard to their hearing status, and reminds us that parent-child perceptions do not always completely match. Deaf adolescents are increasingly facing challenges related to peer acceptance, fitting into groups in the face of unclear auditory input in noisy situations, and struggling with their identities as individuals with unique differences compared to their peers (Sheridan, 2008). Substantiating this perspective, interviews with 11 children and adolescents indicates that situations involving hearing peers were often difficult, compounded by limited access to the subtleties and nuances of social interactions (Punch & Hyde, 2011b). However, a more recent study of 33 participants with a mean age of 10.12 (SD = 3.59) who had been implanted prior to age 2 notes that peer acceptance was rated as the least problematic area based on a self-report quality of life questionnaire (Warner-Czyz, Loy, Roland, & Tobey, 2013). This study suggests that long-term use may have a positive impact for socialization purposes, that is, if communication is efficient and the environment is supportive.

Interestingly, in a study of German children aged 6 to 15, participants with cochlear implants noted less satisfaction with their quality of life at school than did those without cochlear implants, while in general both groups did not significantly differ in overall quality of life (Mattejat & Remschmidt, 2006, as cited in Fellinger & Holzinger, 2011). Additionally a study of the psychosocial adjustment of 57 adolescents, with and without cochlear implants, indicated no significant differences in measures of measures of self-perception, satisfaction with life, and loneliness despite some differences in background characteristics (Leigh, Maxwell-McCaw, Bat-Chava, & Christiansen, 2009). Considering that the adolescents without cochlear implants who participated in this study were primarily in schools for deaf students and preferred American Sign Language (ASL), while the adolescents with cochlear implants were primarily spoken-language users and in the mainstream, the results of this study corroborate the findings of Mattejat and Remschmidt (2006, as cited in Fellinger & Holzinger, 2011) with regard to overall similarity in quality of life for those with and without cochlear implants. With reference to school settings, these studies indicate that while overall quality of life may be positive, at least in the German study as well as the Loy et al., (2010) study, domain-specific areas such as those related to the school environment may indicate areas of vulnerability.

Another study (Moog, Geers, Gustus, & Brenner, 2011) reports results indicating strong social skills, friendships with both hearing and deaf peers, and high self-esteem for a sample of 112 adolescents with long-term cochlear-implant use. What is noteworthy is that the authors of this study acknowledge possible sample selection bias, meaning that this sample may not represent the psychosocial characteristics of the entire population of adolescents with long-term use of cochlear implants.

One critical factor in quality-of-life ratings involves quality of communication among family members. One study that focused on deaf adolescents, not necessarily with cochlear implants, finds that youths who stated that they understood

a large part of their parents' expressive communication reported a higher perceived quality of life related to their sense of self, relationships, and environment
as well as being deaf or hard of hearing (Kushalnagar, Topolski, Schick, Edwards,
Skalicky, & Patrick, 2011). Hence, as Moog et al. (2011) show, it is not only the
cochlear implant that affects quality of life but also environmental variables that
support the individual.

Peer Group Concerns

Studies have shown that successful one-on-one peer relationships do not necessarily extend to group situations. A study (Martin et al., 2010) in which 10 implanted preschool children aged 5–6 were observed interacting with each other
within the context of a peer-entry task reveals that interactions were more productive in one-on-one situations than in interactions during which the implanted
child interacted with two hearing peers. This confirms the need for increased attention to targeted interventions that may facilitate group peer interactions, depending on context. Based on an Austrian study of 32 adolescents with cochlear
implants whose parents and teachers were administered the Strengths and Difficulties Questionnaire, findings suggest that this sample did not exhibit emotional
problems, inattention-hyperactivity, conduct problems, and pro-social behavior
more often than a hearing sample (Huber & Kipman, 2011). Interestingly, only the
teacher ratings indicated an increased risk of problems for these peers compared
to hearing peers. In interviews with 24 parents, 15 teachers, and 11 children and
youth with cochlear implants, the consensus was that interactions with hearing
peers were less than ideal (Punch & Hyde, 2011b).

Loneliness has also been researched. Two studies that relied on measures of
loneliness demonstrate roughly equal scores for loneliness among children and
youth with cochlear implants and hearing samples related to the loneliness measures (Leigh et al., 2009; Schorr, 2006). In contrast, Wauters and Knoors (2008) conducted a study of 18 deaf children between 7 and 9 years of age (9 of whom had
cochlear implants) who were in inclusive settings with hearing peers. For both the
deaf and the hearing students, they found that the deaf participants scored lower
on prosocial behavior and higher on socially withdrawn behavior. At this point,
it may be safe to assume that even though loneliness may not significantly differ
on loneliness measures, closer scrutiny may reveal more loneliness, particularly
related to group situations.

Conclusion: Psychosocial Health

Contrary to fears expressed by those who perceive the push toward pediatric
cochlear implantation as problematic for psychosocial development, the data

mentioned here indicate that cochlear implants per se are not necessarily creating maladjusted individuals, although the possibility of frustrating communication situations and problematic social situations does exist (Punch & Hyde, 2011b). Given that research studies tend to involve individuals who have positive perceptions of the implant, Christiansen and Leigh (2002/2005) made a concerted effort to include the parents of children whose experience with the cochlear implant was not necessarily positive in order to obtain a spectrum of perspectives, but to no avail. It is possible to assume that these potential subjects do not readily participate in cochlear implant research projects. Consequently, as mentioned earlier (Moog et al., 2013), the threat of sample bias is present. For example, if children and youth with additional complex issues were included in these studies (see for example Dammeyer [2010]), results have the potential to be more varied. We need to access this population in order to ensure that the goal of optimizing cochlear implant usage is fully realized for those who undergo implantation by targeting appropriate intervention strategies. However, all things considered, supportive environments and individual attributes, including resilience, are factors that are crucial in ensuring positive psychosocial stability (e.g., Zand & Pierce, 2011).

Many of the participants with cochlear implants in the studies mentioned earlier rely on spoken language, thus raising questions about how they label themselves in the deaf-hearing identity domain. It is intriguing that a technological development could have the power to influence one's identity, the sense of who one is. This possibility is explored in the next section.

STUDIES OF IDENTITY

Going back in history to the Old and the New Testaments, as well as to ancient Egypt, Greece, and Rome, deaf persons were identified as people who could not hear, communicated differently, and may or may not have been rejected by the societies in which they lived (Abrams, 1998; Bauman, 2008; Eriksson, 1993; Miles, 2000; Rée, 1999; Van Cleve & Crouch, 1989). Paralleling the rise of education for deaf children during the 1500s was the emergence of Deaf groups who took pride in being part of a Deaf constituency and contradicting those who focused on deficiency and disability (Branson & Miller, 2002; Mottez, 1993; Quartararo, 2008). Subsequently, this process led to the emergence of formal study of the espousal of a Deaf identity, forged particularly through the centralized education of deaf children in residential schools for deaf youngsters. In these schools, deaf children developed and reinforced social relationships with deaf peers, the parameters of which evolved into Deaf cultural ways of being, outside the strictly educational sphere (Burch, 2002; Rée, 1999; Van Cleve & Crouch, 1989).

So, what exactly is a culturally Deaf identity? It has come to mean ways of being that rely on language and thought expressed through visual relationships and markers of signed languages, a key component of which is the use of the eyes in daily interactions. Auditory components of daily living, including the use of spoken language, do not have primacy in the lives of culturally Deaf people, as they do for hearing people.

Not all deaf people assert Deaf culture identities, and not all necessarily organize their lives exclusively on vision. Many spend time exclusively within their hearing society, feel at home using spoken language, and live culturally hearing lifestyles (Leigh, 1999, 2009). These different perceptions of deaf lives have given rise to various theories of deaf identities and how these are internalized. Neil Glickman's (1996) work, based on racial identity development theories, has gained the most traction in terms of understanding how deaf people categorize themselves and at times transition from one identity category to another. Glickman's psychological theory focuses on how oppressed minority groups develop positive identities based on their interactions within both their own group and the majority group. Thus, identities in this case are shaped by the psychological impact of social interactions.

The description of the culturally hearing indicated earlier falls into the first of Glickman's (ibid.) four categories of deaf identities. The second category covers cultural marginality, including those who do not fully identify with or have a sense of belonging to either Deaf or hearing groups. These individuals are further differentiated into two types: The first comprises those with inadequate access to spoken or signed languages, a situation that exacerbates social and psychological marginality in terms of confusion regarding identity, poorly differentiated understanding of oneself and others, and difficulties with self-regulation of emotions and behavior; the second consists of linguistically competent individuals who are in the process of actively exploring their sense of identity as culturally hearing or Deaf or, as Hintermair (2008) contends, those who are comfortable with nonaffiliation.

Identification as culturally Deaf, also described as *immersion,* constitutes another category. Deaf identity and Deaf culture are uncritically embraced. These individuals often fit the prototypical type of deaf person: They are fluent in ASL or another native signed language; they typically marry a deaf spouse, work within the Deaf world, and socialize primarily with other Deaf people. The last category, bicultural, comprises those individuals who can integrate the values of both Deaf and hearing cultures and comfortably navigate in either one as the situation demands. Multiple studies indicate that this latter group appears on average to be the most optimally adjusted psychosocially (Cornell & Lyness, 2004; Hintermair, 2008; Jambor & Elliott, 2005).

How do people gravitate toward these identity categories and internalize who they are? And what impact does this have on one's identity? Social connections and exposure to specific groups are clearly factors that figure prominently in how deaf individuals formulate their identities. Shared and effective ways of communicating with one's peers, whether via spoken or signed languages, will facilitate the strengthening of social relationships and of social identities with specific groups for which they have an affinity. This has been demonstrated by a variety of studies investigating social relationships (e.g., Bat-Chava, 2000; Kluwin & Stinson, 1993). Generally, individuals who prefer signed languages will identify with those who also use their language, while those who prefer spoken language will identify with like-minded peers. Today, more and more deaf and hard of hearing individuals are identifying themselves as bicultural, preferring to gravitate between various social environments and shifting language use as needed.

Maxwell-McCaw and Zea (2011) suggest similarities between new immigrants to the United States navigating between their home culture and the new American culture, and Deaf people navigating between deaf and hearing cultures. Thus, the concept of acculturation provides an additional pathway to understanding how deaf identities evolve, with several factors in addition to social influences that can ultimately shape the process of acculturation to both the Deaf and the hearing cultures. These factors include the level of psychological identification with each culture; the degree of cultural involvement; preferences for one culture or the other; competence in the language used; and knowledge of the cultures. One's process of acculturation to each group can be measured by assessing varying levels of the factors involved in this undertaking. For example, Hintermair (2008), using a German translation of the Deaf Acculturation Scale,[1] finds that those participants who actually preferred to be marginal rather than be defined by either Deaf or hearing cultures actually demonstrated positive psychological resources in facilitating their adjustment. So, in this case, marginalization does not necessarily assume maladjustment. However, a deaf spoken-language user new to Deaf culture and its relevant signed language may be marginal if the individual does not identify fully with hearing peers; but, with increased exposure to the pertinent Deaf cultural ways and increasing mastery of the relevant signed language, that person is said to be acculturating to Deaf culture. This would be indicated through increasingly higher scores for the various factors associated with Deaf acculturation.

Interestingly, for individuals with cochlear implants, a complex constellation of issues related to identity formation comes into play. As the Deaf and the hearing cultures often have contradictory attitudes toward cochlear implants, with the former seeing them as a potential threat to their culture and the latter typically perceiving them as a great advance in enhancing auditory skills and spoken language, the question of what happens to deaf identity formation becomes relevant.

Influence of Cochlear Implants on Deaf Identities

Although the history of cochlear implants described earlier demonstrates how they may play a role in the formation of identity, the focus of the informed consent documents used by cochlear-implant centers is primarily on medical, audiological, communicative, and educational aspects, giving short shrift to acculturation issues. For example, a study by Berg, Ip, Hurst, and Herb (2007) indicates that fewer than half of the 121 centers in the United States that responded to a nationwide survey included information on Deaf culture and ASL. This finding strongly suggests a bias toward developing hearing-acculturated identities on the part of cochlear implant centers. Whether this hearing-acculturated identity continues to be paramount depends in large part on the individual attributes of the children themselves, the environments in which they are reared, the level of exposure to signing environments, and the availability and quality of their social interactions with their hearing and deaf peers.

A number of studies indicate that parents tended to be practical regarding the necessity of using signed languages, particularly prior to implantation, and as needed postimplantation (Christiansen & Leigh, 2002/2005; Paludneviciene & Leigh, 2011; Watson, Hardie, Archbold, & Wheeler, 2008; Yoshinaga-Itano, 2006; Zaidman-Zait, 2008). At the very least this sets the stage for possible bilingualism and biculturalism in cochlear implant users in contrast to the typical expectation that children with cochlear implants are automatically perceived as hearing acculturated and relying only on spoken language.

Wald and Knutsen's (2000) study of 45 deaf adolescents with and without cochlear implants not surprisingly found that hearing identity as measured by Glickman's (1996) Deaf Identity Development Scale (DIDS) was more frequently endorsed by adolescents with cochlear implants than by those without implants, possibly in part because of improved socialization with their hearing peers. Interestingly, both groups similarly endorsed cultural marginality, immersion, and particularly the bicultural category. This similarity reappears in the Most, Weisel, and Blitzer (2007) study, in which 115 deaf Israeli adolescents participated, only 10 of whom had cochlear implants. Specifically, the two groups did not significantly differ in terms of DIDS classifications. The authors consider the endorsement of a bicultural identity for these implanted adolescents as allowing for the potential to benefit from this technology without having to sacrifice the Deaf experience.

Similar results were noted in the U.S. questionnaire study of 57 deaf adolescents with and without cochlear implants mentioned earlier (Leigh et al., 2009), with results from the Deaf Acculturation Scale (DAS; Maxwell-McCaw & Zea, 2011) indicating that most of the adolescents with cochlear implants were in mainstream settings and affirmed having a hearing-oriented identity. Yet, the number of cochlear-implanted adolescents having a bicultural identity was similar to those in deaf settings, again affirming the salience of this identity for the cochlear-implant group. In their study of 107 adolescents with long-term cochlear-implant use, Moog et al. (2011) find that identification was with either the hearing community (32%) or with both the deaf and the hearing communities (thereby identifying as bicultural, 38%).

Most of the 14 adolescent and young adult cochlear-implant users interviewed in the Christiansen and Leigh (2002/2005) study reported viewing themselves as deaf and had deaf friends while also desiring contact with both deaf and hearing peers. In an interview study with younger children, Preisler, Tvingstedt, and Ahlström (2005) noted that these children saw the implant as a natural part of their lives and used signed as well as spoken languages. This suggested to the authors that the children would be better off claiming bicultural identities. In a semistructured questionnaire interview study involving 29 British adolescents aged 13 to 16 with cochlear implants who were in both mainstreamed and specialized educational settings, it was found that most of the participants were flexible in terms of communication mode (spoken and signed languages) and endorsed a deaf identity that was neither culturally Deaf nor strongly hearing (Wheeler, Archbold, Gregory, & Skipp, 2007).

Overall, children and adolescents with cochlear implants tend to affirm either a hearing-oriented identity or a bicultural identity. These identity choices reflect comfort with what they are and their socialization preferences. It has been noted that increasing numbers of deaf students with cochlear implants attend specialized college programs for deaf students (Brueggemann, 2008; Ladd, 2007). This adds credence to the value attributed to bicultural identities and the need to explore the deaf part of oneself, particularly with regard to entering environments with significant numbers of Deaf peers and communicating with them in ASL. The Deaf community today is more accepting of cochlear implant users and eager to share their culture and language with these individuals.

CONCLUSION

In sum, all of the data presented here suggest that it is time to end the either-or paradigm: either cochlear implantee or culturally Deaf (Hintermair & Albertini, 2005). It is also time to end the perception that cochlear implant users are going to be rejected by culturally Deaf groups. Despite pockets of resistance as mentioned earlier in this chapter, it appears that the fusion approach has some credibility, particularly with evidence of generally positive psychosocial well-being. However, "Research related to deafness appears to lack a systematic and comprehensive framework of proactive psychosocial attributes and tactics that adults who are deaf use to maximize their professional and social potential" (Jacobs, 2010, p. 5). In addition, because school curricula typically do not include the development of proactive psychosocial skills, the psychosocial potential maximization framework could be modified to identify proactive psychosocial attributes and tactics that may work with populations of deaf children and youth (ibid.). This framework consists of eight psychosocial themes, seven of which fall under two thematic categories: internal decisions and external manifestations. Internal decisions, covering the cognitive attributes of desire, goal orientation, and reframing, in turn influence external manifestations, including persistence, goodness of fit, learned creativity, and social ecologies. The eighth—and overarching—theme is control. (See Jacobs, 2010; Jacobs, Brown, & Paatsch, 2012, for further details.) This framework could be utilized to explore strategies that facilitate the positive psychosocial development indicated by many of the studies reported here with the hope of applying these strategies to those children and youth who are struggling with psychosocial and mental health issues.

NOTE

1. See the discussion of an updated Deaf Acculturation Scale in Maxwell-McCaw and Zea (2011).

REFERENCES

Abrams, J. (1998). *Judaism and disability.* Washington, DC: Gallaudet University Press.

Bat-Chava, Y. (2000). Diversity of deaf identities. *American Annals of the Deaf, 145,* 420–428.

Bat-Chava, Y., & Deignan, E. (2001). Peer relationships of children with cochlear implants. *Journal of Deaf Studies and Deaf Education, 6,* 186–199.

Bat-Chava, Y., Martin, D., & Kosciw, J. (2005). Longitudinal improvements in communication and socialization of deaf children with cochlear implants and hearing aids: Evidence from parental reports. *Journal of Child Psychology and Psychiatry, 46*(12), 1287.

Bauman, H.-D. (2008). On the disconstruction of (sign) language in the Western tradition: A Deaf reading of Plato's *Cratylus.* In H.-D. Bauman (Ed.), *Open your eyes: Deaf studies talking* (pp. 127–145). Minneapolis: University of Minnesota Press.

Berg, A., Herb, A., & Hurst, M. (2005). Cochlear implants in children: Ethics, informed consent, and parental decision making. *Journal of Clinical Ethics, 16*(3), 239–250.

Berg, A. L., Ip, S. C., Hurst, M., & Herb, A. (2007). Cochlear implants in young children: Informed consent as a process and current practices. *American Journal of Audiology, 16*(1), 13–28. doi: 10.1044/1059-0889(2007/003)

Blume, S. (1999). Histories of cochlear implantation. *Social Science & Medicine, 49,* 1257–1268.

Boyd, R., Knutson, J., & Dahlstrom, A. (2000). Social interaction of pediatric cochlear implant recipients with age-matched peers. *Annals of Otology, Rhinology, and Laryngology, 109*(Suppl. 185), 105–109.

Branson, J., & Miller, D. (2002). *Damned for their difference: The cultural construction of deaf people as disabled.* Washington, DC: Gallaudet University Press.

Brueggemann, B. J. (2008). Think-between: A Deaf studies commonplace book. In H.-D. Bauman (Ed.), *Open your eyes: Deaf studies talking* (pp. 177–188). Minneapolis: University of Minnesota Press.

Burch, S. (2002). *Signs of resistance: American Deaf cultural history, 1900 to 1942.* New York: New York University Press.

Chmiel, R., Sutton, L., & Jenkins, H. (2000). Quality of life in children with cochlear implants. *Annals of Otology, Rhinology, & Laryngology, 109*(12) (Suppl. 185), 103–105.

Christiansen, J. B., & Leigh, I. W. (2002/2005). *Cochlear implants in children: Ethics and choices.* Washington, DC: Gallaudet University Press.

Christiansen, J. B., & Leigh, I. W. (2011). Cochlear implants and deaf community perceptions. In R. Paludneviciene & I. W. Leigh (Eds.), *Cochlear implants: Evolving perspectives* (pp. 39–55). Washington, DC: Gallaudet University Press.

Cornell, S., & Lyness, K. (2004). Therapeutic implications for adolescent deaf identity and self-concept. *Journal of Feminist Family Therapy, 16,* 31–49.

Dammeyer, J. (2010). Psychosocial development in a Danish population of children with cochlear implants and deaf and hard-of-hearing children. *Journal of Deaf Studies and Deaf Education, 15*(1), 50–58.

Eriksson, P. (1993). *The history of deaf people.* Örebro, Sweden: SIH Läromedel.

Fellinger, J., & Holzinger, D. (2011). Enhancing resilience to mental health disorders in deaf school children. In D. Zand & K. Pierce (Eds.), *Resilience in deaf children* (pp. 169–205). New York: Springer.

Glickman, N. (1996). The development of culturally deaf identities. In N. Glickman & M. Harvey (Eds.), *Culturally affirmative psychotherapy with deaf persons* (pp. 115–153). Mahwah, NJ: Erlbaum.

Hintermair, M. (2008). Self-esteem and satisfaction with life of deaf and hard-of-hearing people: A resource-oriented approach to identity work. *Journal of Deaf Studies and Deaf Education, 13*(2), 278–300.

Hintermair, M., & Albertini, J. (2005). Ethics, deafness, and new medical technologies. *Journal of Deaf Studies and Deaf Education, 10*(2), 185–192.

House, W. E., & Berliner, K. (1991). From idea to clinical practice. In H. Cooper (Ed.), *Cochlear implants: A practical guide* (pp. 9–33). London: Whurr.

Huber, M., & Kipman, U. (2011). The mental health of deaf adolescents with cochlear implants compared to their hearing peers. *International Journal of Audiology, 50,* 146–154.

Huttunen, K., & Välimaa, T. (2010). Parents' views on changes in their child's communication and linguistic and socioemotional development after cochlear implantation. *Journal of Deaf Studies and Deaf Education, 15*(4), 383–404.

Jacobs, P. (2010). Psychosocial potential maximization: A framework of proactive psychosocial attributes and tactics used by individuals who are deaf. *Volta Review, 110*(1), 5–29.

Jacobs, P., Brown, P. M., & Paatsch, L. (2012). Social and professional participation of individuals who are Deaf: Utilizing the psychosocial potential maximization framework. *Volta Review, 112*(1), 37–62.

Jambor, E., & Elliott, M. (2005). Self-esteem and coping strategies among deaf students. *Journal of Deaf Studies and Deaf Education, 10*(1), 63–81.

Kluwin, T., & Stewart, D. (2000). Cochlear implants for younger children: A preliminary description of the parental decision and outcomes. *American Annals of the Deaf, 145*(1), 26–32.

Kluwin, T., & Stinson, M. (1993). *Deaf students in local public high schools: Background, experiences, and outcomes.* Springfield, IL: Charles C. Thomas.

Knutson, J., Boyd, R., Reid, J., Mayne, T., & Fetrow, R. (1997). Observational assessments of the interaction of implant recipients with family and peers: Preliminary findings. *Otolaryngology: Head and Neck Surgery, 117*(3), 196–207.

Kushalnagar, P., Topolski, T., Schick, B., Edwards. T., Skalicky, A., & Patrick, D. (2011). Mode of communication, perceived level of understanding, and perceived quality of life in youth who are deaf or hard of hearing. *Journal of Deaf Studies and Deaf Education, 16*(4), 512–523.

Ladd, P. (2007). Cochlear implantation, colonialism, and Deaf rights. In L. Komesaroff (Ed.), *Surgical consent* (pp. 1–29). Washington, DC: Gallaudet University Press.

Leigh, I. W. (1999). Inclusive education and personal development. *Journal of Deaf Studies and Deaf Education, 4,* 236–245.

Leigh, I. W. (2009). *A lens on deaf identities.* New York: Oxford University Press.

Leigh, I. W., Maxwell-McCaw, D., Bat-Chava, Y., & Christiansen, J. B. (2009). Correlates of psychosocial adjustment in deaf adolescents with and without cochlear implants: A preliminary investigation. *Journal of Deaf Studies and Deaf Education, 14*(2), 244–259.

Loy, E., Warner-Czyz, A., Tong, L., Tobey, E., & Roland, P. (2010). The children speak: An examination of the quality of life of pediatric cochlear implant users. *Otolaryngology: Head & Neck Surgery, 142*(2): 247–253.

Marche, S. (2012). Is Facebook making us lonely? *Atlantic.* Retrieved April 24, 2012, from http://www.theatlantic.com/magazine/archive/2012/05/is-facebook-making-us-lonely/308930/

Martin, D., Bat-Chava, Y., Lalwani, A., & Waltzman, S. (2011). Peer relationships of deaf children with cochlear implants: Predictors of peer entry and peer interaction success. *Journal of Deaf Studies and Deaf Education, 16*(1), 108–120.

Mattejat, F., & Remschmidt, H. (2006). *ILK inventar zur erfassung der lebensqualität bei kindern und jugendlichen: Ratingbogen für kinder, jugendliche und eltern.* Bern: Huber.

Maxwell-McCaw, D., & Zea, M. C. (2011). The Deaf Acculturation Scale (DAS): Development and validation of a 58-item measure. *Journal of Deaf Studies and Deaf Education, 16,* 325–342.

Meserole, R., Carson, C., Riley, A., Wang, N., Quittner, A., Eisenberg, L., … Niparko, J. (2014). Assessment of health-related quality of life 6 years after childhood cochlear implantation. *Quality of Life Research, 23*(2), 719–731.

Miles, M. (2000). Signing in the seraglio: Mutes, dwarfs, and jesters at the Ottoman Court 1500–1700. *Disability and Society 15*(1), 115–134.

Moog, J., Geers, A., Gustus, C., & Brenner, C. (2011). Psychosocial adjustment in adolescents who have used cochlear implants since preschool. *Ear & Hearing, 32*(Suppl. 1), 75S–83S.

Most, T., Wiesel, A., & Blitzer, T. (2007). Identity and attitudes towards cochlear implant among deaf and hard of hearing adolescents. *Deafness and Education International, 9*(2), 68–82.

Mottez, B. (1993). The deaf-mute banquets and the birth of the deaf movement. In J. Van Cleve (Ed.), *Deaf history unveiled* (pp. 27–39). Washington, DC: Gallaudet University Press.

Nicholas, J., & Geers, A. (2003). Personal, social, and family adjustment in school-aged children with a cochlear implant. *Ear & Hearing, 24,* 69S–80S.

Niparko, J., & Wilson, B. (2000). History of cochlear implants. In *Cochlear implants: Principles and practices* (pp. 103–107). Philadelphia: Lippincott Williams & Wilkins.

Paludneviciene, R., & Leigh, I. W. (Eds.). (2011). *Cochlear implants: Evolving perspectives.* Washington, DC: Gallaudet University Press.

Percy-Smith, L., Cayé-Thomasen, P., Gudman, M., Jensen, J., & Thomsen, J. (2008). Self-esteem and social well-being of children with cochlear implant compared to normal-hearing children. *International Journal of Pediatric Otorhinolaryngology, 72,* 1113–1120.

Percy-Smith, L., Jensen, J., Cayé-Thomasen, P., Thomsen, J., Gudman, M., & Lopez, A. (2008). Factors that affect the social well-being of children with cochlear implants. *Cochlear Implants International, 9*(4), 199–214.

Percy-Smith, L., Jensen, J., Josvassen, J., Jonsson, M., Andersen, J., Samar, C., Thomsen, J., & Pedersen, B. (2006). *Ugeskr Laeger, 168*(33), 2659–2664.

Preisler, G., Tvingstedt, A., & Ahlström, M. (2005). Interviews with deaf children about their experiences using cochlear implants. *American Annals of the Deaf, 150*(3), 260–267.

Punch, R., & Hyde, M. (2011a). Social participation of children and adolescents with cochlear implants: A qualitative analysis of parent, teacher, and child interviews. *Journal of Deaf Studies and Deaf Education, 16*(4), 474–493.

Punch, R. & Hyde, M. (2011b, January). Communication, psychosocial, and educational outcomes of children with cochlear implants and challenges remaining for professionals and parents. *International Journal of Otolaryngology, 4*, 1–10. Article ID 573280, http://doi:10.1155/2011/53280

Quartararo, A. (2008). *Deaf identity and social images in nineteenth-century France.* Washington, DC: Gallaudet University Press.

Rée, J. (1999). *I see a voice.* New York: Metropolitan Books.

Roan, S. (2009, August 3). Cochlear implants open deaf kids' ears to the world. *Los Angeles Times.* Retrieved August 3, 2009, from http://articles.latimes.com/2009/aug/03/health/he-deaf-children3

Schindler, R. A. (1999). Personal reflections on cochlear implants. *Annals of Otology, Rhinology, and Laryngology, 108*(Suppl. 177), 4–7.

Schorr, E. (2006). Early cochlear implant experience and emotional functioning during childhood: Loneliness in middle and late childhood. *Volta Review, 106*(3), 365–379.

Schorr, E., Roth, F., & Fox, N. (2009). Quality of life for children with cochlear implants: Perceived benefits and problems and the perception of single words and emotional sounds. *Journal of Speech, Language, and Hearing Research, 52*(1), 141–152.

Sheridan, M. A. (2008). *Deaf adolescents: Inner lives and lifeworld development.* Washington, DC: Gallaudet University Press.

Van Cleve, J., & Crouch, B. (1989). *A place of their own: Creating the Deaf community in America.* Washington, DC: Gallaudet University Press.

Venail, F., Vieu, A., Artieres, F., Mondain, M., & Uziel, A. (2010). Educational and employment achievement in prelingually deaf children who receive cochlear implants. *Archives of Otolaryngology: Head & Neck Surgery, 136*(4), 366–372.

Wald, R., & Knutsen, J. (2000). Deaf cultural identity of adolescents with and without cochlear implants. *Annals of Otology, Rhinology, & Laryngology 12*(2) (Suppl. 185), 87–89.

Warner-Czyz, A., Loy, B., Roland, P., & Tobey, E. (2013). A comparative study of psychosocial development in children who receive cochlear implants. *Cochlear Implants International, 14*(5), 266–275.

Warner-Czyz, A., Loy, B., Roland, P., Tong, L., & Tobey, E. (2009). Parent versus child assessment of quality of life in children using cochlear implants. *International Journal of Pediatric Otorhinolaryngology, 73*, 1423–1429.

Watson, L., Hardie, T., Archbold, S., & Wheeler, A. (2008). Parents' views on changing communication after cochlear implantation. *Journal of Deaf Studies and Deaf Education, 13*(1), 104–116.

Wauters, L., & Knoors, H. (2008). Social integration of deaf children in inclusive settings. *Journal of Deaf Studies and Deaf Education, 13*(1), 21–36.

Wheeler, A., Archbold, S., Gregory, S., & Skipp, A. (2007). Cochlear implants: The young people's perspective. *Journal of Deaf Studies and Deaf Education, 12*(3), 303–316.

Yoshinaga-Itano, C. (2006). Early identification, communication modality, and the development of speech and spoken language skills. In P. Spencer & M. Marschark (Eds.), *Advances in the spoken language development of deaf and hard-of-hearing children* (pp. 298–327). New York: Oxford University Press.

Zaidman-Zait, A. (2008). Everyday problems and stress faced by parents of children with cochlear implants. *Rehabilitation Psychology, 53*(2), 139–152.

Zand, D., & Pierce, K. (2011). *Resilience in deaf children: Adaptation through emerging adulthood.* New York: Springer.

Deaf Populations

Part 2

7

Self-Esteem of Deaf and Hard of Hearing People in Cyprus and Greece

Katerina Antonopoulou
Kika Hadjikakou
Maria Charalambous

Self-esteem is defined as one's overall evaluation or appraisal of one's own worth (Rosenberg, 1979; Smith & Mackie, 2007). Self-esteem encompasses beliefs (e.g., "I am competent," "I am worthy") and emotions such as triumph, despair, pride, and shame. Similarly, one's self-esteem is based on the ratio between perceived competence and one's aspirations in at least one specific area of life that one considers important (Harter, 1990). Discrepancies between perceived and actual competence, as acknowledged by oneself and other important people, put one at risk for impairment in self-esteem. Both deaf and hearing women have been found to describe self-esteem in conceptually equivalent terms, with most women in each group referring to the notion of "capability" (Holte & Dinis, 2001).

Self-esteem has been found to affect the cognitive, emotional, and social aspects of human development (Campbell & Lavallee, 1993). Several studies have revealed that deaf and hard of hearing individuals have lower self-esteem than hearing people (Bat-Chava, 1994; Mulcahy, 1998; Schlesinger, 2000; Weisel & Kamara, 2005). In addition, "several aspects might affect self-esteem and well-being, such as vocational dissatisfaction, frustration in attempts at communication, and social rejection" (Weisel & Kamara, 2005, p. 59). Thus research on the self-esteem of deaf and hard of hearing people should take into consideration the circumstances in which they grew up or their current conditions in relation to their communicative and acceptance experiences, overall psychosocial potential, and general satisfaction with life (Hintermair, 2007). Previous studies have proposed a number of factors that may influence the self-esteem of deaf and hard of hearing people, including parents' hearing status, the mode of communication at home, educational experiences prior to college, acculturation, the age of onset of deafness, the severity of hearing loss, and subjective assessments of well-being (Bat-Chava, 1993; Jambor & Elliott, 2005; Maxwell-McCaw, 2001).

In the qualitative research conducted by Sheppard and Badger (2010) and Hadjikakou and Nikolaraizi (2008), the influence of early family communication patterns on later self-esteem was revealed. Deaf participants indicated that they felt isolated as children, given the lack of communication between them and other family members at home; their parents could not sign with them. Parents' hearing status as well as methods of communication within families have an impact on deaf and hard of hearing people's self-esteem (Crowe, 2003; Desselle, 1994; Sheppard & Badger, 2010). Children of deaf parents were found to have greater self-esteem than children of hearing parents (Crowe, 2003; Woolfe & Smith, 2001), probably because deaf parents serve as effective role models for their deaf and hard of hearing children. Also, deaf and hard of hearing people whose parents used sign language with them had greater self-esteem than did those whose parents preferred oral methods (Crowe, 2003; Desselle, 1994).

A qualitative study of classroom communication barriers (especially in inclusive settings) that might affect the self-esteem of deaf and hard of hearing people has found that deaf women were more likely to report education as a factor in self-esteem enhancement, with language and communication as additional critical components (Holte & Dinis 2001). Other studies have examined the connection between acculturation and self-esteem and/or self-worth. In fact, "group identification is deemed one of the most important factors leading to positive self-esteem among deaf people" (Jambor & Elliott, 2005, p. 67). A number of studies have found that people who described themselves as having a bicultural or deaf identity had greater self-esteem than those with a hearing or marginal identity (Bat-Chava, 2000; Hintermair, 2007; Maxwell-McCaw, 2001; Weinberg & Sterrit, 1986).

THE CONTEXT OF CYPRUS

The history of deaf education in Cyprus began in 1953, when the first school for deaf children was established in Nicosia as a result of a collective effort by the Rotary Club at Nicosia, the Municipal Corporation of Nicosia, and the Government of Cyprus. Until 1987, deaf and hard of hearing students had been attending the school for deaf students exclusively. Then, with the implementation of the (113[1]99) Special Education Law in 1999, the majority of these children in Cyprus (95%) began being educated in general (oral training) schools, either individually or in self-contained classes, with or without special support. The school for deaf children nowadays operates mainly as a provider of various services and programs for children and adults with hearing impairment, along with their families.

Universal hearing screening has been in place in Cyprus since 2005, and almost all newly identified deaf and hard of hearing children receive cochlear implants and are orally educated (Lampropoulou & Hadjikakou, 2010).

During the last few years, the growing Deaf community has developed an active role with a number of Deaf clubs established in various towns on the island. These include the Club for Young People with Hearing Loss, which was founded in 2010 in Nicosia and focuses mainly on the entertainment and welfare of young deaf people. Deaf clubs were founded in Limassol and Larnaca in 1995, with a combined membership of nearly 250. All of these clubs (except the one in Larnaca, which rents its space) have their own premises and are open at least twice a week. They, as well as the Pancyprian Association of the Deaf and the Athletic Union for the Deaf, are all under the joint jurisdiction of the Cyprus Deaf Athletic Federation, which was established in 1997 and deals with athletic issues related to Deaf people, and the Cyprus Federation for the Deaf, which was founded only in 2004 and focuses on social and legal issues related to Deaf people and the Deaf culture. In April 2006, due to great efforts made by the Cyprus Federation of the Deaf, Cyprus Sign Language was recognized by the Cyprus Parliament (Law 66[I] 2006) as being equivalent to Greek; the Deaf community is now advocating for the implementation of bilingual education (Hadjikakou & Nikolaraizi, 2011).

THE CONTEXT OF GREECE

The history of formal deaf education in Greece began in 1923 with the establishment of the first school (Lampropoulou, 1994), with more schools (both private and public) for deaf children established throughout the country. Until 1982, the education of deaf and hard of hearing students fell mostly under the auspices of the Ministry of Health and Welfare and was offered in segregated, oral settings. From 1980 to 1990 a movement of parents, professionals, and people with disabilities demanded the integration of students with disabilities into general education. In 1984 the Ministry of Education, through new legislation (PL. 1566/85), undertook the responsibility of the education of children with disabilities, including deaf youngsters, and developed special day schools and integrated units within the nation's regular schools. Some full-time inclusion programs in general classes were also offered to a limited number of students. In 2000 Greek Sign Language (GSL) was recognized by the Special Education Law (PL. 2817/2000) as the primary language of Deaf people; teachers were required to be fluent in GSL regardless of the method they chose to communicate with their deaf and hard of hearing students. In 2008, legislation (PL. 3699) was passed to implement bilingual education (Lampropoulou & Hadjikakou, 2010).

Members of the Greek Deaf community participate actively in decision-making bodies, demanding quality education for deaf and hard of hearing children. The first Greek Association of the Deaf was established in 1948. Today, 19 Deaf organizations throughout Greece are all under the umbrella of the Greek Federation of the Deaf. In 1983 the Theater of the Deaf of Greece was established. Furthermore, in 1989, the Hellenic Athletic Federation of the Deaf was established and assumed responsibility for the development of the athletic activities of Deaf people (Hadjikakou & Nikolaraizi, 2011).

THE AIM OF THE PRESENT STUDY

To develop data on the self-esteem and cultural identity of deaf and hard of hearing adults in Cyprus and Greece, the current study explored the link between these features, including possible differences, as a function of specific demographic factors such as age of onset of deafness, type of schooling, and mode of communication at home. More specifically, the present study sought to answer the following questions:

- What is the level of self-esteem of deaf and hard of hearing adults in Cyprus and Greece?
- What kind of cultural identity have deaf and hard of hearing adults in Cyprus and Greece developed?
- Is there a link between self-esteem and cultural identity?
- With regard to their level of self-esteem and cultural identity, do the deaf and hard of hearing adults who were born deaf and those who lost their hearing during their childhood exhibit any significant differences?
- With regard to their level of self-esteem and cultural identity, do the deaf and hard of hearing adults who were educated in general schools and those who attended special schools for deaf children exhibit any significant differences?
- With regard to their level of self-esteem and cultural identity, do the deaf and hard of hearing adults who communicate using signs at home and those who communicate orally exhibit any significant differences?
- Does their preferred identification contribute to deaf and hard of hearing individuals' self-esteem?

METHOD

Participants and Procedure

Eighty-four deaf and hard of hearing individuals from Cyprus ($n = 39$) and Greece ($n = 45$) participated in the study. Of these, 66.7% were between 18 and 37 years of age (44% male and 56% female). Participants were recruited through personal contact and invitations issued by local associations for deaf and hard of hearing individuals and their families from Nicosia in Cyprus and Athens in Greece.

During scheduled home visits, participants were informed of the purpose of the study, and confidentiality procedures were explained. Then, they were given instructions on how to complete the questionnaires and given an opportunity to do so.

Instruments

Demographic characteristics and cultural identity were measured using the questionnaire devised by Jambor and Elliott (2005). It is a self-report questionnaire consisting of short scales measuring cultural identification (identification with the deaf community, identification with the hearing community, and bicultural identification) and demographic variables such as age, gender, mode of communication, onset of deafness, and type of schooling. The group identification scale comprises 22 items on a four-point Likert-type scale (1 = completely untrue, 2 = somewhat untrue, 3 = somewhat true, 4 = completely true). Participants were asked to indicate the extent to which they agreed with the statements that were related to group membership or contact with other people in general (e.g., "Relationships with other deaf people are important to me"). Higher in-group identification scores indicated that the participant strongly identified with the in-group. A total score was calculated as the mean rating across items on the scale. Cronbach's alpha for the entire scale in this study was .67, which is considered satisfactory.

Self-esteem was measured using the Rosenberg Self-Esteem Scale (Rosenberg, 1979). This scale comprises 10 items that are scored using a four-point Likert-type scale from "strongly disagree" (1) to "strongly agree" (4); half of the items were scored in the reverse direction, and the total mean score was calculated for an indication of the individuals' reported self-esteem. A high score indicates high self-esteem. Cronbach's alpha for the scale in this study was .79, which is considered satisfactory.

RESULTS

Descriptive Data

Of the participating deaf and hard of hearing adults, 56% stated that they were born with hearing loss, while the remaining 44% said that they acquired loss of hearing at some point in their childhood. Of the participants 75% were deaf, and 25% hard of hearing. Many of the participants reported that they had been educated exclusively at a special school for deaf students (41.5%) and that they communicated orally at home (51.2%). Table 1 presents the participants' demographic profile.

Table 2 shows the mean ratings given by participants responding to the items on the cultural identity and self-esteem scale, with significantly higher scores obtained for bicultural identity preference [$F_{(2, 166)} = 3.75$, $p < 0.05$].

TABLE 1.   Demographic Characteristics of the Participants ($N = 84$)

	F	%
Onset of deafness		
congenital (born with hearing loss)	47	56
acquired (during childhood)	37	44
Severity		
severe	63	75
moderate	21	25
Type of schooling		
special school for deaf students	34	41.5
mainstream school with special needs unit	10	10.9
mainstream school	27	32.1
both mainstream and special school	13	15.5
Communication at home		
oral communication	43	51.2
oral communication and signs	31	36.9
sign language	10	10.9

TABLE 2.   Mean Ratings for Preferred Identifications and Self-Esteem of Participants ($N = 84$)

	Mean	SD	Minimum	Maximum
identification with the deaf community	3.07	0.74	1.13	4
identification with the hearing community	3.04	0.45	2	3.8
bicultural identity	3.26	0.69	1.5	4
global self-esteem	3.13	0.46	2	4

Differences in Self-Esteem and Preferred Identifications as a Function of Demographic Parameters

In order to examine possible differences in self-esteem and cultural identity as a function of the age of onset of deafness, the type of education received, and the primary mode of communication at home, t-tests and one-way ANOVAs were performed. With regard to deaf identification, the results showed a significant difference between the participants who reported that they were born deaf and hard of hearing and those who reported that they had lost their hearing in early childhood. Congenitally deaf participants achieved a higher score in the identification with the deaf community scale than later-deafened individuals ($t_{82} = 2.33$, $p < 0.05$). However, this difference could not be explained by variability in the age of onset of hearing loss, as this variable was not found to be related to identification with deaf people ($\chi^2 = 17.32$, $p > 0.05$). The participants who reported having attended general schools appeared to identify more strongly with hearing people (mean = 3.25) than did those who attended special schools (mean = 2.88) [$F_{(3, 72)} = 3.58$, $p < 0.05$]. This difference in preferred identification could be explained by variability in the type of education received during childhood and adolescence, as this was found to be related to identification with hearing people ($rho = 0.243$, $p < 0.05$). Finally, individuals who reported primarily oral communication at home tended to have a stronger hearing identity (mean = 3.16) than those who used sign language (mean = 2.66) [$F_{(2, 80)} = 5.31$, $p < 0.01$]. This difference could be explained by variability in the mode of communication at home, as this variable was positively correlated with hearing identity ($rho = 0.308$, $p < 0.001$). No other significant difference in preferred identification between groups was found. Additionally, there was no significant difference in self-esteem between groups. This indicates that variability in the age of onset of hearing loss, the type of education received during childhood, and the mode of communication at home do not lead to any differentiation in self-esteem in this particular sample of deaf and hard of hearing individuals.

Preferred Identification Predicting Self-Esteem

In a preliminary analysis, in order to identify links between self-esteem and preferred identification for the total sample, Spearman correlations (rho) were performed. A statistically significant positive correlation between self-esteem and identification with the deaf community ($rho = .268$, p = 0.014) was found, suggesting that deaf and hard of hearing individuals who identify more strongly with the deaf community tend to develop greater self-esteem. No other significant correlation was found.

Given the correlation between self-esteem and identification with the deaf community, a simple linear regression was conducted to determine whether identification with the deaf community may be a good predictor of the deaf and hard of hearing participant's self-esteem. Thus, self-esteem was used as the response variable, and identification with the deaf community was the explanatory variable. One significant but rather reduced positive effect emerged on deaf and hard of hearing adults' self-esteem for identification with the deaf community, accounting for only 5% of the predicted change in variance ($B = .158$, $\beta = .255$, $R^2_{adjusted} = .054$,

$t = 2.387, p < 0.05$). The results indicate that identification with the deaf community is a significant but not very strong predictor of deaf and hard of hearing individuals' self-esteem in this study.

In addition, correlational analyses between self-esteem and all of the identification variables were conducted for different groups according to the age of onset of hearing loss, education type, and mode of communication at home (Tables 3, 4, and 5). One positive significant correlation was found between self-esteem and identification with the deaf community in the congenitally deaf group, and another positive correlation between self-esteem and hearing identity in the later-deafened group (see Table 3). Identification with the deaf community was found to make a significant contribution to congenitally deaf individuals' self-esteem ($B = .476, \beta = .628, R^2_{adjusted} = .381, t = 5.416, p < 0.001$), whereas identification with the hearing community was not found to contribute to the self-esteem of later-deafened participants.

Self-esteem was positively related to identification with the deaf community in those participants who attended a special school for deaf children, whereas in the group of both general and special education receivers, self-esteem correlated positively with identification with the hearing community (Table 4). The regression coefficients indicated that participants' preferred identification had a strong positive effect on self-esteem in both the special education group ($B = .669, \beta = .678, R^2_{adjusted} = .443, t = 5.219, p < 0.001$) and the combination group (general and special education) ($B = .521, \beta = .566, R^2_{adjusted} = .245, t = 2.061, p < 0.05$).

Finally, self-esteem was positively related to bicultural identity in those participants whose preferred mode of communication at home is both oral and signs, whereas in the group of sign-only users, self-esteem relates positively to identification with the deaf community (Table 5). The regression coefficients indicated that participants' preferred identification had a strong positive effect on self-esteem in the oral and signs-only group ($B = .348, \beta = .490, R^2_{adjusted} = .214, t = 3.029, p < 0.01$).

TABLE 3.   Correlations between Identification Preference and Self-Esteem for Congenitally Deaf and Later-Deafened Groups Separately

	Global Self-Esteem	
	Born with Hearing Loss ($n = 47$)	Hearing Loss During Childhood ($n = 37$)
Preferred identification	*rho*	*rho*
deaf	.605**	−.179
hearing	.273	.336*
bicultural	.215	.042

*$p < 0.05$, **$p < 0.01$

TABLE 4. Correlations between Identification Preference and Self-Esteem for the Four Type-of-Education Groups

	Global Self-Esteem			
	Special School For Deaf Students ($N = 34$)	Mainstream School with Unit for Special Education Needs ($N = 10$)	Mainstream School ($N = 27$)	Mainstream and Special School ($N = 13$)
Preferred identification	rho	rho	rho	rho
deaf	.683**	.294	.111	.355
hearing	.255	−.368	.316	.675*
bicultural	.085	−.572	.151	.534

*$p < 0.05$, **$p < 0.01$

TABLE 5. Correlations between Identification Preference and Self-Esteem for the Three Mode-of-Communication Groups

	Global Self-Esteem		
	Oral Communication ($N = 43$)	Oral Communication & Signs ($N = 31$)	Sign Language ($N = 10$)
Preferred identification	rho	rho	rho
deaf	.322	.144	.674*
hearing	.311	.403	−.333
bicultural	−.029	.517**	−.156

*$p < 0.05$, **$p < 0.01$

CONCLUSION

The present study sought to explore the correlations between self-esteem and cultural identity, as well as possible relationships among self-esteem, cultural identity, and selected demographic factors (age of onset, schooling, communication mode) in deaf and hard of hearing adults in Cyprus and Greece.

The results indicate that deaf and hard of hearing adult participants showed positive self-esteem overall and tended to prefer a bicultural identity. The finding of a positive correlation between self-esteem and identification with the deaf community is consistent with previous empirical data suggesting that deaf and bicultural identities in deaf and hard of hearing people correlate with high self-esteem, whereas those with hearing or marginal identities tend to have lower self-esteem (Bat-Chava, 2000; Hintermair, 2007; Weinberg & Sterrit, 1986).

The findings for the subgroups of deaf and hard of hearing participants, defined by the age of onset of hearing loss, education type, and mode of communication at home are obviously interrelated as it appeared that variations in preferred identification contribute significantly to self-esteem in specific deaf and hard of hearing subgroups. For example, we found that deaf identification contributes significantly to the prediction of high self-esteem in the congenitally deaf group or the special education group, while bicultural preference contributes positively to the self-esteem of those deaf and hard of hearing individuals who use both oral language and signs in their communication; on the other hand, hearing identification can predict self-esteem in the mixed-education subgroup. These findings are in line with previous data attesting to the contribution of group identification to self-esteem among deaf and hard of hearing people (Jambor & Elliott, 2005), as well as the moderating role of several contributing factors such as the mode of communication or type of education (Bat-Chava, 1993, 1994; Hadjikakou & Nikolaraizi, 2007, 2008).

In terms of deaf and hard of hearing individuals' preferred identification and demographic characteristics, our findings indicated that individuals who were born deaf tended to identify better with the Deaf community; in contrast, those who reported receiving instruction in general educational settings or communicating orally with parents and other family members tended to identify better with the hearing community. These results are in accordance with previous research data that have shown that attending mainstream schools (where the majority of pupils are hearing), while at the same time having an opportunity to interact and socialize with deaf peers, can be beneficial to deaf children, who can learn how to function in and cope with the hearing world (Kluwin, 1999). Moreover, previous evidence suggests that deaf and hard of hearing children who grow up in a family environment where communication is oral learn to develop a hearing identity, but the impact of this mode of communication at home on the child's psychosocial development is not always positive (Jambor & Elliott, 2005).

It is a fact that in the years to come more and more deaf children will be integrated into mainstream schools (Hyde & Power, 2004; Lampropoulou & Hadjikakou, 2010; Moores, 2001) and will develop hearing, marginal, or bicultural identities, whereas fewer deaf and hard of hearing children will attend schools for deaf students and will consequently develop deaf identities. However, what emerges from our study, and is also supported by other researchers (Bat-Chava, 2000; Maxwell-McCaw, 2001), is that culturally deaf and bicultural individuals have greater self-esteem than those with culturally hearing identities. Thus, policymakers and stakeholders all around the world, as also suggested by Hadjikakou and Nikolaraizi (2007), should take into account the following factors in order to ensure the development of healthy identities within the deaf school population: (a) exposure of deaf and hard of hearing children to the deaf culture within the mainstream school in the morning (e.g., through sign language courses, the employment of deaf adults, or the establishment of bilingual programs) and through participation in the deaf clubs' activities in the evenings; (b) encouragement of deaf and hard of hearing children attending mainstream schools to develop good manual and oral communicative skills that will enable them to immerse themselves successfully in both the hearing and the deaf world in their adult lives. Finally, our findings have important implications also for parents' awareness of the importance of exposing their children to deaf role models and to sign language in order to promote their children's pride in both (hearing and deaf) cultures and communities (Hadjikakou & Nikolaraizi, 2007).

REFERENCES

Bat-Chava, Y. (1993). Antecedents of self-esteem in Deaf people: A meta-analytic review. *Rehabilitation Psychology, 38,* 221–233.

Bat-Chava, Y. (1994). Group identification and self-esteem of deaf adults. *Personality and Social Psychology Bulletin, 20,* 494–502.

Bat-Chava, Y. (2000). Diversity of deaf identities. *American Annals of the Deaf, 145,* 420–428.

Campbell, J. D., & Lavallee, L. F. (1993). Who am I? The role of self-concept confusion in understanding the behavior of people with low self-esteem. In R. F. Baumeister (Ed.), *Self-esteem: The puzzle of low self-regard* (pp. 3–20). New York: Plenum.

Crowe, T. V. (2003). Self-esteem among deaf college students: An examination of gender and parents' hearing status and signing ability. *Journal of Deaf Studies and Deaf Education, 8,* 199–206.

Desselle, D. D. (1994). Self-esteem, family climate and communication patterns in relation to deafness. *American Annals of the Deaf, 139,* 322–328.

Hadjikakou, K., & Nikolaraizi, M. (2007). The impact of personal educational experiences and communication practices on the construction of deaf identity in Cyprus. *American Annals of the Deaf, 152*(4), 398–414.

Hadjikakou, K., & Nikolaraizi, M. (2008). The communication experiences of adult deaf people within their family during childhood in Cyprus. *Deafness and Education International, 10*(2), 60–79.

Hadjikakou, K., & Nikolaraizi, M. (2011). Deaf clubs today: Do they still have a role to play? *American Annals of the Deaf, 155*(5), 605–617.

Harter, S. (1990). Processes underlying adolescent self-concept formation. In R. Montemayor, G. R. Adams, & T. P. Gullotta (Eds.), *From childhood to adolescence: A transitional period?* Newbury Park, CA: Sage.

Hintermair, M. (2007). Self-esteem and satisfaction with life of deaf and hard-of-hearing people. A resource-oriented approach to identity work. *Journal of Deaf Studies and Deaf Education, 13*(2), 278–300.

Holte, M. C., & Dinis, M. C. (2001). Self-esteem enhancement in Deaf and hearing women: Success stories. *American Annals of the Deaf, 146*(4), 348–354.

Hyde, M., & Power, D. (2004). Inclusion of deaf students: An examination of definitions of inclusion in relation to findings of a recent Australian study of deaf students in regular classes. *Deafness and Education International, 6,* 82–99.

Jambor, E., & Elliott, M. (2005). Self-esteem and coping strategies among deaf students. *Journal of Deaf Studies and Deaf Education, 10*(1), 63–81.

Kluwin, T. (1999). Co-teaching deaf and hearing students: Research on social interaction. *American Annals of the Deaf, 144,* 339–344.

Lampropoulou, V. (1994). The history of deaf education in Greece. In C. J. Erting, R. C. Johnson, D. L. Smith, & B. D. Snider, (Eds.), *The Deaf Way* (pp. 239–249). Washington, DC: Gallaudet University Press.

Lampropoulou, V., & Hadjikakou, K. (2010). An examination of deaf history in Greece and in Cyprus: Investigating determinant factors for its development. *L1: Educational Studies in Language and Literature, 10*(1), 41–56.

Maxwell-McCaw, D. L. (2001). Acculturation and psychological well-being in deaf and hard-of-hearing people. Doctoral dissertation, George Washington University. *Dissertation Abstracts International, 61* (11B), 6141.

Moores, D. F. (2001). *Educating the deaf: Psychology, principles and practices* (5th ed.). Boston: Houghton Mifflin.

Mulcahy, R. T. (1998). Cognitive self-appraisal of depression and self-concept: Measurement alternatives for evaluating affective states. Unpublished doctoral dissertation, Gallaudet University.

Rosenberg, M. (1979). *Conceiving the self.* New York: Basic Books.

Schlesinger, H. S. (2000). A developmental model applied to problems of deafness. *Journal of Deaf Studies and Deaf Education, 5*(4), 349–361.

Sheppard, K., & Badger, T. (2010). The lived experience of depression among culturally Deaf adults. *Journal of Psychiatric and Mental Health Nursing, 17,* 783–789.

Smith, E. R., & Mackie, D. M. (2007). *Social psychology* (3rd ed.). New York: Psychology Press.

Weinberg, N., & Sterritt, M. (1986). Disability and identity: A study of identity patterns in adolescents with hearing impairments. *Rehabilitation Psychology, 31,* 95–102.

Weisel, A., & Kamara, A. (2005). Attachment and individuation of deaf/hard-of-hearing and hearing young adults. *Journal of Deaf Studies and Deaf Education, 10*(1), 51–62.

Woolfe, T., & Smith, P. K. (2001). The self-esteem and cohesion to family members of deaf children in relation to the hearing status of their parents and siblings. *Deafness and Education International, 3*(2), 80–96.

8

Public Health of Deaf People

Johannes Fellinger

Defined by the World Health Organization in 1986 as a state of well-being in the physical, mental, and social areas of life,[1] health is a gift but also a great responsibility. Individuals must take care of their health. It is society's responsibility to establish a basis on which to promote health, as documented in the WHO Bangkok Charter for Health Promotion in 2005.[2] Public health is the social and political concept of improving physical well-being, prolonging life, and improving the quality of life among whole populations through a variety of forms of health intervention, such as health promotion and disease prevention.[3]

Health inequities for deaf people have been reflected in editorial comments such as "Deafness might damage your health" and "The health of deaf people: Communication breakdown" in *The Lancet* (2012),[4] which accurately express the problems of public health care for deaf people. In the same volume, the article "Mental health of deaf people" ends with a revision of the slogan "No health without mental health" and emphasizes that deaf people cannot get help for their mental health problems when barriers restrict access to general health care.[5] Health inequities for deaf people are of increased interest in the field of public health research.[6, 7, 8] Deaf patients report fear, mistrust, and frustration in health-care settings.[9] A global survey carried out in 2011 by the World Federation of the Deaf Health Resources Initiative shows that 80% of Deaf leaders worldwide report significant problems in accessing health care.[10]

Although public awareness of these inequities for Deaf people is increasing, the problem itself is not new. Influenced by my father's deafness and negative experiences in the health-care system (e.g., hearing comments like "The patient is deaf and dumb . . . impossible to take his/her history"), in 1991 I established a small psychiatric outpatient clinic at the hospital of St. John of God in Linz. When it became apparent that physical problems and social issues needed to be tackled as well, the clinic expanded in 1993 to offer multidisciplinary services for Deaf people according to the WHO's holistic approach to health.

Other health centers for deaf persons (HCD) were founded in Vienna and
Salzburg in 1999 and in Graz (Styria) in 2008; the HCD in Vienna and Graz are
integrated into hospital run by the order of St. John of God, while the one in
Salzburg is part of a state hospital).

DATA FROM PATIENTS AT THE LINZ
HEALTH CENTER FOR DEAF PEOPLE

Upper Austria has approximately 1.4 million inhabitants. According to prevalence
rates of 0.07 to 0.1 %[11,12] approximately 988 citizens are prelingually deaf. In 2011
nearly three-quarters (724 persons) of these individuals were treated at the HCD
(see Table 1) in Linz (the capital city of Upper Austria).

In 2011, out of the 724 patients who visited the HCD in Linz, 252 used both
medical and social services, 342 had appointments only with a general practitioner, and 130 had appointments only with social workers or psychologists.

PATIENT CHARACTERISTICS

From 1991 to 2011 the Linz HCD had nearly 1,900 Deaf patients, 85% of whom
were prelingually deaf. These patients and clients were evenly distributed among
all age groups.

In 1993–1994 352 Deaf patients were interviewed. Approximately 60% of the
Deaf patients were married or in a steady relationship. About 10% of the patients'
children had a hearing impairment. Approximately 67% of the patients reported
having only friends with a hearing impairment, while 67% reported being active
members of a Deaf club. Seventy percent reported being content with their job and
having no problems with their hearing coworkers; however, 25% would rather

TABLE 1.   Demographics and HCD Users

	Linz (since 1991)	Vienna (since 1999)	Graz (since 2008)
federal, state, and total population	Upper Austria 1,411,041	capital city 1,692,067	Styria 1,207,588
estimated number of deaf inhabitants per federal state	988	1,184	845
number of HCD patients since inception of HCD	1,900	1,229	429

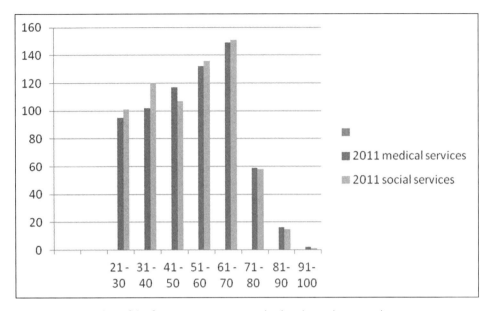

FIGURE 1.   Number of deaf patients receiving medical and social services by age.

find different employment. The Deaf patients earned approximately 23.5% less than the general working population.[13]

HEALTH-RELATED DATA

From the early years of providing medical services to Deaf patients, the HCDs were able to collect information about the clients' medical issues. At that time, 40% of all patients who had diabetes mellitus or pathological glucose-tolerance diabetes were diagnosed at the HCD, and 45% were diagnosed with high blood pressure. Surgery was needed by 10% of the patients.

As a result of available medical treatment, symptoms of diseases such as hypertonia were perceptibly improved. After the fourth year of routine checkups, high-risk patients showed major improvements and high treatment compliance.

The HCDs' findings from health checkups during the first year were compared to data on the hearing population in Austria. Results show that, compared to hearing people, the Deaf more often felt nervous and stressed. They also suffered from back pain and joint pain and complained about stomach and intestinal problems three times as often as hearing people and about headaches six times as often (see Table 2).

Additionally, middle-aged Deaf men (40 and over) and younger adult women (20–30 years of age) tended to experience more nervousness or feel stressed and overwhelmed. Furthermore, data on the Deaf patients' mental health were compared to those on the hearing population in Germany. The comparison showed

TABLE 2. Comparison of the Most Frequent Subjective Mental and Somatic Complaints during Health Checkups

Complaints	Deaf N = 352	Hearing N = 273	χ^2 df = 1	p
mental and/or somatic complaints	244 (69.3%)	150 (54.9%)	$\chi^2 = 13.63$	< 0.001
nervous, scared, overburdened, overwhelmed	244 (69.3%)	123 (45.1%)	$\chi^2 = 37.34$	< 0.001
back pains	159 (45.2%)	69 (25.3%)	$\chi^2 = 26.28$	< 0.001
intestinal complaints	115 (32.7%)	26 (9.5%)	$\chi^2 = 26.79$	< 0.001
cardiopulmonary complaints	107 (30.4%)	60 (22.0%)	$\chi^2 = 5.57$	< 0.05
constipation	81 (23.0%)	28 (10.3%)	$\chi^2 = 17.37$	< 0.001
headaches	64 (18.2%)	9 (3.3%)	$\chi^2 = 33.04$	< 0.001

that psychiatric conditions such as schizophrenia, addiction, and alcoholism, as well as mood disorders such as bipolar disorder, were as common in Deaf as in hearing populations.

Even though Deaf and hearing patients showed comparable percentages of psychiatric diagnoses for schizophrenia, addiction/alcoholism, mood/bipolar disorders, this same study also showed that Deaf patients were more frequently diagnosed with somatoform disorders than the hearing population in Germany (see Table 3).[14, 15]

After comparing patient data, the following question arose: How are not only the HCDs' clientele but the Deaf population in general doing in terms of stress and quality of life? A comprehensive study that utilized a large community sample of Deaf people (n = 236) attempted to answer that question in 2003 and 2004. Internationally approved research instruments (World Health Organization's Brief Quality of Life WHOQOL-BREF, 12-Item General Health Questionnaire GHQ-12 and the Brief Symptom Inventory [BSI]) were translated into Austrian Sign Language for this study.[16] The results showed a significantly poorer quality of life for the physical and psychological domains (p < 0.01) of the Deaf sample than for the general hearing population as measured by the WHOQOL-BREF. In the domain of social relationships, no significant difference was demonstrated. All findings with the GHQ-12 and the BSI showed much higher levels (p < 0.01) of emotional distress among the Deaf participants.[17]

That research project could be carried out only in close cooperation with the Deaf community. A trusting relationship with the HCD had been developed

TABLE 3. Frequency of Selected Mental Disorders: Comparison between HCD Patients and Hearing Patients in Germany (Using Corresponding Data from General Practitioners in Germany)

ICD-10 Categories	Disorder	Amount N (Sum Total = 310)	Percentage	Hearing People in Germany %
F1	mental and behavioral disorders caused by psychotropic substances	18	5.8	6.3
F2	schizophrenia, schizotypal and paranoid disorders	12	3.9	ns
F3	mood disorder	35	11.3	9.3
F4	neurosis, stress, and somatoform disorders	101	32.6	21
F6	personality and behavioral disorder	44	14.2	ns

through the effective support that deaf people experienced at the HCD, the concept of which is described in the next section.

Another research project on quality of life in an elder and middle-aged Deaf community sample showed also the positive effect of social networking between Deaf people.[18]

DESCRIPTION OF THE CONCEPT OF HEALTH CENTERS FOR DEAF PEOPLE IN AUSTRIA

The main objectives of a HCD (health center for the deaf) are as follows:

1. To examine and treat Deaf patients in primary care who are suffering from acute and chronic illnesses, including mental health disorders
2. To offer personalized preventive medicine
3. To take advantage of the medical network (consultants, hospitals) and help adapt hospital offerings (e.g., radiology) to meet the needs of the Deaf patients
4. To support Deaf inpatients' care as well as their treating medical staff (nurses, physicians)
5. To offer high-quality specialized mental health services
6. To provide community health in a broader sense by integrating social work
7. To supply health education for Deaf patients

Structural Prerequisites

- Ideally, an HCD will be affiliated with a general hospital for more readily accessible medical services and inpatient treatments.
- Deaf patients should be able to arrange their appointments via text message, e-mail, fax, or video chat and with appropriate privacy (e.g., giving patients a chance to sign in areas where the communication cannot be observed by others).
- The accessibility of the visual and technical environment for Deaf people will be enhanced, with appropriate lighting, assistive devices, and visual communications and alert systems.

Team

HCDs operate according to a "one-stop" framework, so that Deaf patients have an opportunity to see a number of specialists for medical, psychological, and social issues in one visit. Ideally such specialists would include the following: general practitioner; nurse; psychologist; social worker; sign language interpreter; other pertinent specialists (psychiatrists, linguists); in addition, having Deaf employees is crucial since they ensure the use of visual communication and raise awareness of Deaf culture and perspective needed when treating Deaf patients. Employees in a health center require communication and accessibility skills. They must be fluent

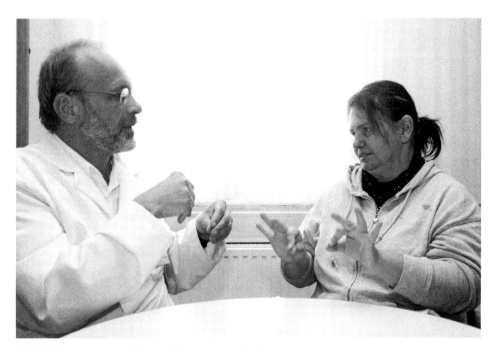

PHOTO 1.   Johannes Fellinger, MD, in a psychiatric setting.

in the national sign language in order to understand the Deaf patients and to make themselves understood. They also need the following expertise:

- Skills in nonverbal communication (visual information, drawings, pantomime) to also provide Deaf people who are not proficient in signed or written language with the information needed
- Awareness of the communication needs of people who are hard of hearing (e.g., providing good lighting conditions to facilitate lipreading, clear articulation)
- Proficiency in using technical equipment that is designed to help people with hearing impairments (amplifier, etc.)
- Understanding the patients' needs and wishes: Employees have to be able to recognize body language indicating cautious rejection, especially in connection with the nodding syndrome. Deaf patients often nod their assent to close a difficult conversation without really understanding the issue that was discussed.

Cultural Awareness

- Knowledge and understanding of Deaf culture and the willingness to immerse oneself in it, including awareness of educational backgrounds and experiences (with special reference to health education), and life situations (work and social conditions). Cultural awareness is expressed in many everyday situations. As employees for instance have to make numerous phone calls during their workday it is of great importance that the Deaf patient is included in the conversation by giving that individual information about the reason for and the content of the call.
- Empowering patients to make their own decisions and to take responsibility for their health.

Ability to Cooperate

- Willingness to be part of an interdisciplinary team: Employees are part of a multidisciplinary network. They have ample opportunity to learn from their coworkers and use this expertise in their doctor-patient relationship.
- Professional cooperation with interpreters and understanding of their profession (positioning, confidentiality, etc.)
- Willingness to cooperate with a Deaf relay interpreter. Often Deaf native speakers understand Deaf patients better and are understood by them more easily in difficult situations.

The Need for Specific Knowledge

- about the health conditions of deaf people
- about the relevant legal framework (antidiscrimination laws, etc.)

IMPLEMENTATION OF THE SEVEN MAIN OBJECTIVES

Objective 1: To Examine and Treat Deaf Patients with Acute and Chronic Illnesses as well as Mental Health Problems and Disorders in Primary Care

Deaf patients who live near the HCD tend to visit it more often with acute medical problems. For those who visit their local general practitioners (GP) in more remote regions it is not rare for the HCD to reach out to get in touch with the GPs to clear up misunderstandings resulting from problems in communication with Deaf patients.

∾

Example: A 56-year-old Deaf man signed to his local general physician about pain in the pectoral area. The GP, thinking the patient was describing bronchitis, prescribed mucolytic drugs. When the patient's medical history was properly taken in sign language at the HCD, it became clear that the problems were caused by an angina pectoris. Further cardiological examinations showed that the patient had coronary vessel disease and needed a bypass operation.

∾

The HCD offers medical services that are usually provided by local general practitioners. House calls, however, can be made only to a limited extent.

An HCD's general practitioner is also required to recognize physical symptoms that point to psychological disorders.

∾

Example: Because of her complaints of stomach pain, a 35-year-old Deaf woman received repeated gastroscopic examinations at an external hospital. After finally obtaining the patient's history, it became clear that the stomachaches started after the woman had been raped. Referred for psychotherapy to help process the trauma, the stomach problems were quickly resolved.

∾

It is particularly important to be able to treat chronic illnesses at the HCD. In dealing with these, patients must receive comprehensive information about the course of treatment in order to follow the instructions accurately. Managing diabetes in Deaf patients is only one of many such examples.

$\sim$

Example: In the course of a preventive checkup by her local general practitioner, a 30-year-old Deaf woman was diagnosed with juvenile-onset
diabetes. Living far from the HCD and due to the language barrier, her
therapy was limited to getting insulin prescriptions. The woman repeatedly developed hypoglycemia. Several times she was found unconscious
by her 9-year-old daughter, who had to call an ambulance. The daughter was traumatized by these incidents. Peaks in the woman's HbA1c
showed that the prescribed long-term management of the diabetes was
insufficient. After having attended a 3-week intensive education program
designed for deaf people with diabetes as well as well as ongoing treatment monitoring by the HCD, the woman's diabetes stabilized, and her
health improved. The daughter was also relieved of the stress of dealing
with repeated crises.

$\sim$

Objective 2: Personalized Preventive Medicine

In the health centers for deaf persons, preventive checkups consist not only of a
medical exam but health education and pertinent patient information as well.

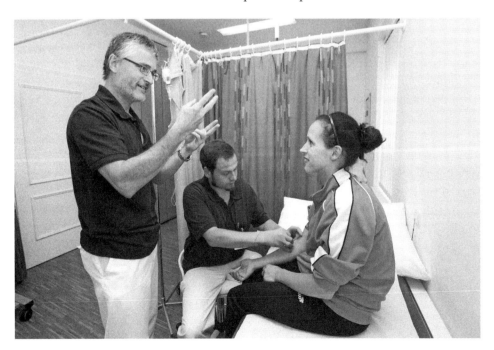

PHOTO 2.   Wolfgang Schatzlmayr, MD, in a medical service.

The regular preventive health checkup (*Gesundenuntersuchung*) is the heart of all preventive medicine, giving the physician an opportunity to evaluate the general state of the patient's health and psychosocial condition, as well as, for Deaf patients, to inquire about the factors associated with deafness. Furthermore, the physician can also inquire into family, genetic and vaccinations history as well as about general health hazards such as smoking and drinking habits, working and living conditions. Following a special questionnaire, the physician asks the patient about their complaints. After that the physician clinically examines the patient (general state of health) and takes a blood sample (bloodcount, liver parameter, kidney parameter, electrolyte, lipids, blood sugar, uric acid, inflammation parameter, thyroid parameter) and urine sample.

Furthermore, patients are encouraged to visit specialists for regular, routine checkups according to the latest medical standards (e.g., gynecological checkups for sexually mature women every year, mammograms for women aged 40 and older every year or every other year, preventive gastroscopies for patients aged 50 and older, and prostate checkups for men. Patients are also referred to ophthalmologists for basic checkups to recognize risk factors and decreased vision well in advance. Patients who are at risk of suffering from glaucoma are advised to have ophthalmological checkups, including measuring intraocular pressure, at least every other year starting when they turn 19. When patients turn 65, it is recommended that they have their vision and intraocular pressure checked annually.

In addition, patients are advised to have annual dental exams. The general practitioner also trains the patients in preventive routine checkups that they can do on their own, such as monthly breast examinations for women, monthly testicular examinations for men, and monthly inspection of one's skin for moles.

The health center also puts great emphasis on informing patients of measures they can take to live a healthy life. Patients can avail themselves of information about a healthy diet and exercise as well as about mental hygiene, such as stress and conflict management. Support in dealing with issues concerning one's work environment, relationship problems, isolation, and so on is also available. To provide information that is adapted to the Deaf patients' needs, the health center's psychologists, social workers, and medical staff work closely together.

Furthermore, secondary and tertiary prevention of chronic illnesses is crucial. Complications and risks caused by diseases such as diabetes, hypertension, and hyperlipidemia can be reduced when the patient sees a physician for regular checkups. The health center also offers individual and group counseling (stays in health and therapy centers) for degenerative illnesses of the musculoskeletal system, incontinence, obesity, and nicotine dependence.

Objective 3: Cooperation with the Hospital's Departments and Specialists

The HCDs' role within a general hospital setting is to facilitate the use of the hospital's expertise and resources on behalf of Deaf patients, ranging from the use of sign language interpreters to communicate with specialists in various disciplines and with the consent of the patient to sharing medical information between HCD staff and hospital staff.

∼

Example: A rheumatologist and the health center's general practitioner jointly treat patients suffering from a rheumatic disease by seeing the patient at the same time.

∼

Nevertheless, when specialists prescribe treatments, the general practitioner at the HCD often needs to explain these to the patient in detail. In many cases it takes extra time to discuss important therapeutic steps with deaf patients, such as how to take their drugs or how to monitor and take notes about their micturition.

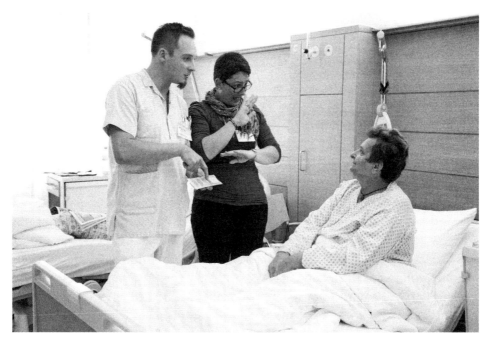

PHOTO 3. Maria Bonis interpreting during a hospital examination.

∾

Example: A Deaf woman suffering from varicose veins consulted a hospital's surgical department, whose consulting surgeon recommended surgery and support stockings. Due to time pressure he did not explain the use of the stockings. When the patient asked the interpreter how to use them, she stated that she did not know but offered to schedule an appointment with the health center's physician. The HCD physician was able to respond to the patient's questions and concerns about how to use the stockings.

∾

Objective 4: Inpatient Care

When a Deaf patient needs to stay in a hospital, the HCD makes sure that a sign language interpreter is on hand during the admissions process, will generally visit these patients daily during their stay, and also be present at discharge. During the hospital stay HCD staff members are available to facilitate communication between hospital staff and the Deaf patient by providing sign language interpreters, as well as discussing the course of their disease and treatment instructions, such as the need to have an empty stomach before a gastroscopy. When a patient is discharged from the hospital, an interpreter is present at the discharge interview. If needed, the HCD's general practitioner discusses the findings with the patient afterward.

Objective 5: Specialized Mental Health Service

By becoming integrated into the HCD, psychiatric and psychological services become more easily accessible, particularly since Deaf—like hearing—patients tend to avoid these services, perhaps because they feel more stigmatized.

Crisis intervention is a crucial resource. The unexpected nature of crises and the need to provide prompt assistance pose a challenge to already busy staff, but this service remains a priority for Deaf patients, as it is for hearing patients. Prompt and accessible crisis intervention can significantly influence the consequences for subsequent health and social care and for finding appropriate solutions more effectively within the field of mental health. Crisis situations arise unexpectedly most of the time and therefore cannot be planned. However, in a crisis it is important for Deaf clients to have prompt and expert help since it can significantly affect their health and social network. Often simply talking about the issues helps to unburden the clients. This makes it possible for them to look to the future and helps them find solutions.

Psychologists and other mental health experts offer medium- and long-term psychological, psychotherapeutic, and psychiatric counseling and treatment. General therapy goals include the improvement of the clients' self-efficiency and the competent utilization of their social network.[19]

The health centers for deaf persons also offer group counseling. For instance, assertiveness training for Deaf teenagers has proven to be of great success. For Deaf people who are admitted to inpatient care in a psychiatric hospital, the HCDs also provide interpreting services.

Objective 6: Community Health in a Broader Sense: Integrated Social Work

Medical issues can also be complicated by psychosocial issues, necessitating the intervention of social workers.

∾

Example: A 24-year-old Deaf man is pale and extremely underweight and has kidney problems. His HCD physician learns that the patient does not have enough money to pay his heating bill. The patient is referred to the HCD social worker, who can help him apply for financial aid.

∾

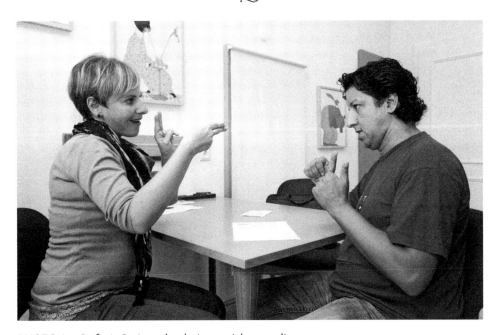

PHOTO 4. Stefanie Breiteneder during social counseling.

Other examples of social counseling include supporting Deaf patients and clients (as well as hard of hearing persons and persons with cochlear implants) and their relatives regarding interpersonal, social, or community issues.

Compared to the hearing population, the Deaf have limited access to information or informal contacts; therefore social counseling is a way to provide information adapted especially to the needs of the clients.

Group and individual counseling sessions aim at preventing, as well as treating problems ranging from supporting Deaf patients and clients in situations in which they encounter communication barriers to advising them on complex issues such as the following:

- Counseling and assistance in their daily life (e.g., family, independent living skills)
- Family and relationship problems
- Finances (e.g., debt counseling, applications for subsidies)
- Living arrangements (e.g., contact with housing associations with respect to renting an apartment)
- Information on new technology
- Problems related to old age
- Support in dealing with issues concerning work (e.g., finding new employment and maintaining existing employment contracts) and employment-related issues (this area is addressed by a separate unit in Linz, where the staff members visit Deaf people at their workplaces)

The social counseling service plans, implements, coordinates, monitors, and evaluates the services offered to the Deaf patients and clients and adapts these services to meet their needs. In this context the cooperation with the health centers' multiprofessional team of physicians, nurses, psychologists, and therapists, as well as the link to other institutions such as public authorities, custodians, and aid agencies, are of the utmost importance.

~

Example: A 65-year-old Deaf woman with limited cognitive abilities had hip-replacement surgery. Her treating staff (i.e., physicians, nurses) were concerned about discharging her to live on her own since she has no contact with relatives and no social safety net. During her stay in the hospital, the hospital's social worker and cross-over care staff registered the patient for a nursing home, applied for care allowance, and arranged for temporary in-home care in the meantime. Furthermore, they applied to the court to appoint a custodian and regularly visited the patient in the hospital and then at home. Within the health center they closely cooperated with other experts (nurse, physician, senior patient therapy center, mobile care). Due to the Deaf patient's mildly limited cognitive abilities, counseling takes more time. However, as a result of the multiprofessional cooperation, the patient's quality of life is significantly improved.

≈

In spite of the complex and varied issues, the social and psychological services need to be easily accessible. Patients are counseled at the health center and at home. Personal support and assistance as well as home visits enable patients to better understand the context and content of the counseling services.

≈

Example: Youth welfare services intervene after a report of abuse in a family with deaf parents and four hearing children aged 2–8. The service funds 12 hours a week of intensive and accessible family care, which is coordinated by the health center's social workers and includes access to a wide range of services, such as family and mental health counseling, medical care, and speech therapy. With this comprehensive support, parenting skills were significantly improved, and the children were able to stay with their parents.

≈

The patients' autonomy and participation are of the utmost importance. On a daily basis the social workers try to connect with their patients and clients and establish mutual trust.

Objective 7: Health Education and Specific Programs

Individual health education takes place primarily after medical checkups. Most often the patients are given important information in the form of pictures or short notes that they can take home. Specific health issues are also discussed in group settings, such as exercises for those who suffer from back pain, losing weight without a diet, incontinence training, parent counseling, and nicotine withdrawal. Once a year the health center for Deaf persons hosts an event that focuses on a specific health topic. Talks are given in Austrian Sign Language, and the participants who attend from throughout Austria have ample opportunity to discuss the relevant issues.

Furthermore, the health center also provides information leaflets that are adapted to the needs of Deaf individuals (e.g., stress, abuse, high blood pressure).

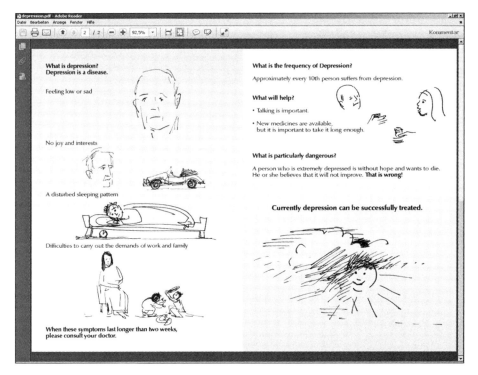

FIGURE 2.   Depression as an example.

FUNDING

Austria consists of nine federal states, and each citizen has compulsory health insurance, thus providing guaranteed medical care. However, the federal states are separately responsible for implementing support measures for people with disabilities; therefore, the funding priorities of the HCD in Vienna, Linz, Salzburg, and Graz may vary considerably.

For instance, Upper Austria passed an equal opportunities act stipulating that people who are Deaf, have a hearing impairment, or suffer from similar communication problems are legally entitled to demand-oriented services, such as those offered by the HCD. The extra time needed when providing medical and social services for Deaf people and the target groups mentioned above is not covered by Austria's general federal health insurance but by the Austria social welfare system. So the total costs are carried by two systems, 85% by the Austria social welfare system and 15% by the Austria's general federal health insurance. However, it is important to emphasize that the HCD is not the only source of medical care available to Deaf persons. They are entitled to arrange for a sign language interpreter for an appointment with a doctor of their choice. The incurred costs for the interpreting services are also borne by Upper Austria's social welfare.

Economic Aspects

Analysis of data from the HCD in Vienna, Linz, and Graz yielded the following suggested model of a specialized, full-time health center offering medical, social, and psychological services. The model is designed for a population of one million people, with a Deaf population of 700–1000 people[20] half of whom live within a 40-minute commute to the center (Table 4).

Every year, treatment per deaf patient per year costs an average of 630 euros. Borne by Upper Austria's medical insurance and welfare departments (about 15%), this sum includes primary care from the general practitioner, nurse, psychologist, and social worker. The additional costs for sign language interpreters or signing staff accompanying Deaf patients to hospital departments are included, though inpatient treatment costs are not. The only figure to compare these with are the costs per patient only at the patient's local general practitioner (124 euros for an average patient in Austria, who sees a GP 6.5 times a year, as the database from the Upper Austria Health Insurance 2011 shows).

In 2011, 594 patients consulted the general practitioner of the health center for Deaf persons in Linz, while an average colleague treating hearing people saw approximately 2,300 patients in the same period of time. As both are working full time (the GP at the HCD only for deaf people and the GP running a typical ordination with hearing patients), one could deduce that providing treatment that is adapted to the Deaf patients' needs is four times more time consuming than treating hearing patients.

It has to be borne in mind, however, that Deaf patients tend to consult a general practitioner closer to their homes for minor ailments, such as a sore throat, and travel to the health center for more severe health issues.

TABLE 4.   Model of a Specialized, Full-Time Health Center Offering Medical, Social, and Psychological Services

Employees	
1 PU = 40 hours/week	1 PU general practitioner
	1.5 PU nurse
	0.7 PU psychologist
	1.25 PU social worker
	1 PU secretary
personnel costs, including 20% infrastructure	380,000 euros
patients per year	600 patients
treatment costs per patient per year	630 euros
number of consultations per patient per year	10 consultations

PU = personnel unit

Apart from the outpatients, the general practitioner and the nurse also tend to Deaf patients who receive inpatient care in the adjoining hospital. The health center practitioner and nurse also cared for a total of 126 Deaf inpatients over 874 days the respective patients stayed in hospital in 2011.

Since Deaf patients have limited access to information about health, providing education about health prevention is a major goal of the health center. Prevention focuses on a high-risk group and is therefore very effective and reduces health-care costs in the long run.[21] Out of the 594 Deaf patients seen in 2011, 136 came to the health center in Linz for annual, routine checkups, which means that one in four patients used preventive care.

Direct services by a physician fluent in Austrian Sign Language also has an economic advantage when compared to the costs that are incurred when arranging for freelance sign language interpreters. Even if an appointment is perfectly coordinated, the cost for a freelance interpreter ranges from at least 90–120 euros in a medical setting. By comparison, a medical consultation at the HCD (medical treatment and barrier-free communication) costs 60 euros.

The sign language interpreters employed by the health centers for deaf persons are able to plan their appointments much more efficiently; therefore the costs

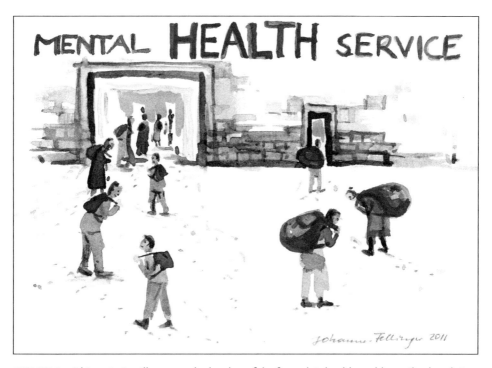

FIGURE 3.   This painting illustrates the burden of deaf people's health problems (backpacks) and the "narrow" access to health care for Deaf people, and the role of the HCD. Reprinted from J. Fellinger, D. Holzinger, & R. Pollard. (2012, March 17). Mental health of deaf people. *Lancet*, *379*, 1037–1044. www.thelancet.com).

can be reduced by two-thirds. Because of the cooperation with the health center's other professionals, the interpreters are able to prepare for appointments much more thoroughly since background information on their patient-client is at hand. When patients have follow-up questions after a doctor's appointment, the sign language interpreters can make use of their network by referring the patient back to the health center's general practitioner and helping them schedule an appointment if necessary. In this way optimal patient care is provided.

SUMMARY AND DISCUSSION

Research findings point to inequities in access and a significant incidence of stress-related disorders. An HCD for Deaf people, as described here, addresses the two major inequities that Deaf people face when accessing health care. On the one hand, consumer-friendly access to health care is provided; on the other hand, focused and consumer-centered health care reduces the numerous risk factors Deaf people have to cope with.

CONCLUSION

Article 25 of the UN Convention on the Rights of Persons with Disabilities draws public attention to the right to enjoy the highest attainable standard of health without discrimination.[22] Moreover, obtaining health care in a trustful relationship based on barrier-free communication and respect for Deaf culture can be regarded as a basic right of Deaf people.

Deaf associations are called upon to join forces with NGOs and governmental authorities to implement their rights in promoting health care in a Deaf-friendly way. It was the Deaf community who, after having experienced treatment at the HCD in Linz, successfully campaigned for HCDs in Vienna, Salzburg, and Graz.

ACKNOWLEDGMENT

I thank Wolfgang Schatzlmayr, Stefanie Breiteneder, Manuela Gusenleitner, and Alexandra Mayer-Weinreich for their support in writing this chapter.

NOTES

1. World Health Organization (1986), http://www.who.int/about/definition/en/print.html
2. World Health Organization (2005), http://www.who.int/healthpromotion/conferences/6gchp/hpr_050829_%20BCHP.pdf

3. World Health Organization (1998), *Health Promotion Glossary.* Retrieved April 14, 2010, from http://www.who.int/healthpromotion/about/HPG/en/

4. Alexander, A., Ladd, P., & Powell, S. (2012, March 17), Deafness might damage your health. (The health of deaf people: Communication breakdown. Editorial.) *Lancet, 397,* 979–981.

5. Fellinger, J., Holzinger, D., & Pollard, R. (2012, March 17), Mental health of deaf people. *Lancet, 379,* 1037–1044.

6. Barnett, S., Klein, J. D., Pollard, R., Q. Jr., Samar, V., Schlehofer, D., Starr, M., et al. (2011), Community participatory research to identify health inequities with deaf sign language users. *American Journal of Public Health,* 101(12): 2235–2238.

7. Barnett, S., McKee, M., Smith, S. R., & Pearson, T. A. (2011). Deaf sign language users, health inequities, and public health: Opportunity for social justice. *Preventing Chronic Disease, 8*(2): A45.

8. Deaf Health, http://deafhealth.org.uk/

9. Steinberg, A., Barnett, S., Meador, H. E., Wiggins, E., & Zazove, P. (2006). Health care system accessibility: Experiences and perceptions of deaf people. *Journal of General Intern Medicine, 21,* 260–266.

10. World Federation of the Deaf, http://www.wfdeaf.org/

11. Mitchell, R. E. (2006). How many deaf people are there in the United States? Estimates from the Survey of Income and Program Participation. *Journal of Deaf Studies and Deaf Education, 11,* 112–119.

12. Bubbico, L., Rosano, A., & Spagnolo, A. (2007). Prevalence of prelingual deafness in Italy. *Acta Otorhinolaryngol Ital, 27,* 17–21.

13. Fellinger, J., Holzinger, D., Schoberberger, R., & Lenz, G. (2005). Psychosoziale Merkmale bei Gehörlosen: Daten aus einer Spezialambulanz für Gehörlose. *Nervenarzt, 76*(1), 43–51.

14. Ibid.

15. Linden, M., Mayer, W., Achberger, M., Herr, R., Helmchen, H., & Benkert, O. (1996). Psychische Erkrankungen und ihre Behandlung in Allgemeinarztpraxen in Deutschland. *Nervenarzt, 67,* 205–215.

16. Fellinger, J., Holzinger, D., Dobner, U., Gerich, J., Lehner, R., Lenz, G., et al. (2005). An innovative and reliable way of measuring health-related quality of life and mental distress in the deaf community. *Social Psychiatry and Psychiatric Epidemiology, 40,* 245–250.

17. Fellinger, J., Holzinger, D., Dobner, U., Gerich, J., Lehner, R., Lenz, G., et al. (2005). Mental distress and quality of life in a deaf population. *Social Psychiatry and Psychiatric Epidemiology, 40,* 737–742.

18. Gerich, J., & Fellinger, J. (2011). Effects of social networks on the quality of life in an elder and middle-aged deaf community sample. *Journal of Deaf Studies and Deaf Education, 17*(1), 102–115.

19. Fellinger et al., Mental distress.

20. Bubbico, Rosano, & Spagnolo, Prevalence of prelingual deafness in Italy.

21. Cohen, J. T., Neumann, P. J., & Weinstein, M. C. (2008, February 14). Does preventive care save money? Health economics and the presidential candidates. *New England Journal of Medicine, 358,* 661–663. http://www.nejm.org/doi/full/10.1056/NEJMp0708558

22. UN Convention on the Rights of Persons with Disabilities. (2006). Retrieved April 27, 2011, from http://www.un.org/disabilities/convention/conventionfull.shtml 19 OÖ Gebietskrankenkasse, HVB-Berichte, E-Card Statistik 2011, FälleUmsatz_AS400.mbd, http://www.oegkk.at

9

Quality of Life of Latino Deaf and Hard of Hearing Individuals in the United States

Poorna Kushalnagar
Melissa Draganac-Hawk
Donald L. Patrick

Research on deaf and hard of hearing Latinos living in the United States shows that this population is rapidly growing and indicates disparities in education and health for this understudied group. The term *Latino* is the grassroots alternative to US government statistical data that use *Hispanic* as a racial/ethnic category and is used accordingly in this chapter. In 2010, about 16.3% of the general population was Latino, up from 12.5% in 2000 (US Census Bureau, 2004, 2011). According to the National Center for Children in Poverty (2011), nearly 65% of all Latino children live in low-income households (Addy, Engelhardt, & Skinner, 2013).

From the standpoint of Bronfenbrenner's ecological model (1979), children's development and perceived quality of life are influenced not only by the family system but also by the other important resources with which the child and family interact (e.g., schools, communities). Youth quality of life (YQoL) can be defined as adolescents' sense of how their lives are going overall as well as their feelings about themselves, their relationships with others, and the opportunities and obstacles that arise in their social and cultural milieu (Edwards et al., 2002; Patrick et al., 2002). This concept can be applied to adolescents from diverse backgrounds regardless of their age, gender, culture, any physical disabilities, and socioeconomic status.

Given the challenges faced by Latino children who are deaf or hard of hearing—growing up in a low-income family, navigating both native Spanish and mainstream English languages, as well as American Sign Language (Delgado, 2001)—the likelihood of a negative impact on their development and perceived quality of life increases. A child who is deaf or hard of hearing may try to accommodate the family's primary communication system by learning to speech-read or lip-read Spanish; the family may resort to using home-based signs that they create for simple words or sentences. Communication in this manner tends to be restricted to topics essential to daily life and precludes discussion of more abstract or complex subjects, an accommodation of sorts that becomes problematic as the child gets older and expects greater access to information. Moreover, "barriers and obstacles such as communication, poverty, discrimination and low self-esteem are more often the crucial reasons for lack of perseverance" (Delgado, 2001, p. 16). Although one could surmise that these factors should be addressed in mental health services that are available and accessible to youths who are deaf or hard of hearing, little systematic information has been collected on the important components of perceived quality of life for these youth. Rarely have they been asked about their lifelong management of issues, both intrinsic and extrinsic, that are affected by their hearing loss.

One can predict that when the language of deaf or hard of hearing youth is different from that used by their parents at home (such as Spanish), the result can be a negative impact on their perceived quality of life. The aim of the current qualitative study, conducted in 2008 and 2009, was to describe the factors that influence perceived quality of life from the perspective of the young people who are deaf or hard of hearing. This critical first step was undertaken in order to develop a conceptually appropriate measure of youth quality of life for these individuals (Patrick et al., 2011) that can be used in interventions or programs to promote healthy development in this cohort.

By conducting qualitative interviews with deaf or hard of hearing Latino youths from Spanish-speaking homes, this study aimed to facilitate an understanding of the relationship between language differences at home, at school, and in the community and the perceived quality of life for this population. This information should help school administrators and staff to work more effectively with deaf and hard of hearing youths and their parents to improve and maintain a positive youth quality of life related to being deaf or hard of hearing and in general.

METHOD

Qualitative interviews were conducted to determine recurrent issues and generate items for a new measure of youth quality of life for young people who are deaf or hard of hearing (YQoL-DHH; Patrick et al., 2011). Qualitative interviews conducted in 2008 and 2009 investigated youths' perceptions of how being deaf or hard of hearing affected the quality of life at home, at school, and in the community. Thematic analyses were used to identify the important QoL issues relevant to this group.

This chapter discusses data from a small subset of 11 deaf and hard of hearing youths who reported spoken Spanish as their family's primary language at home. Because the number of participants in this subpopulation is small, the qualitative data from Latino deaf and hard of hearing children were used only to provide a descriptive summary of key QoL issues that are specific to this subpopulation.

Sampling and Participants

Eleven Latino deaf and hard of hearing youth aged 11–18 years of age were recruited through mainstream public schools with and without special programs for them, day/residential schools for deaf students, clinics, and organizations of parents who have deaf and hard of hearing children. A majority of these participants attended schools for deaf students, while the remainder attended mainstream schools with or without services for individuals who are deaf or hard of hearing.

Approval for this research with human subjects was obtained from the University of Washington–Seattle and the University of Colorado–Denver. For this study, hearing loss was operationalized as a parent-reported level of hearing loss (mild, moderate, moderate-severe, severe, profound), and the sample was selected to represent a broad range of hearing loss in order to obtain diverse perspectives on QoL among deaf or hard of hearing young people with a variety of communication preferences and educational backgrounds.

The youth were approached with regard to participating in the research project as "expert informants" to help design a questionnaire to assess adolescents' thoughts and feelings about their QoL. Screening telephone or videophone interviews were conducted in English, Spanish, or ASL with the parents of the prospective youths. When the youths were identified as being eligible to participate in the study, parental consent and youth assent were then explained over the phone and later obtained in person (for in-person interviews) or by mail (for videophone interviews) prior to conducting the qualitative interviews.

Interview Setting and Procedure

We conducted in-depth interviews with the participants on how being deaf or hard of hearing affects their lives. Each 1-hour interview took place in person when possible or via videophone when not. The participants and their parents were reminded of the need for the young people's conversation to be private and for the videophone to be in an area with no other persons present. Audio recorders or video recorders were used to produce a transcript of the interview. For videophone interviews with participants and interviewers who sign, either webcam software with built-in recording or a videophone with a DVR recording device was used to capture both interviewer and participant data for transcription.

The interview began after the interviewer explained the interview process and obtained the youth's permission to record the interview. Individual interviews were conducted by one of six members of the research team, all of whom were experienced in qualitative interviewing. Participants whose primary language was ASL or English-like signing were interviewed by two researchers who are fluent signers.

The semistructured interview included a series of questions about the participants' perspectives on how, if at all, being deaf or hard of hearing affected their quality of life at home, at school, and in the community. Respondents could also introduce relevant themes (e.g., cultural topics) into their narratives that were not included in the initial interview protocol.

The deaf or hard of hearing interviewees were invited to generally discuss their lives, including cultural values, goals, and expectations, in relation to their peers. Specific probes were used to illuminate stage-salient contexts for the participants, including home, school, work, and community (Bronfenbrenner, 1979), how they believed their lives were affected by having a hearing loss in today's society, and how they perceived being deaf or hard of hearing. Interviewees were recruited until sufficient data were obtained with minimal new or different information.

A "grounded theory" approach guided the data analysis of the interviews and focus groups (Glaser & Strauss, 1967). Grounded theory, which is derived from the sociological theory of symbolic interactionism (Blumer, 1969), is used to model phenomena about which little is known (in this case, the QoL of youth who are deaf or hard of hearing).

ANALYSIS

Two Deaf researchers who were highly fluent in ASL and English were assigned to review and transcribe the videotaped ASL interviews. Transcripts of the audio recorded interviews with the hard of hearing participants were transcribed by a professional transcription service. All of the transcripts were reviewed and coded for themes related to QoL for deaf or hard of hearing youths.

Data-coding strategies included open coding (i.e., assignment of codes to the text based on words or phrases that captured meaning in the data); axial coding (i.e., comparison of open codes to create categories); and selective coding (i.e., the use of frequently occurring axial codes to create core categories, or conceptual model domains) (see Strauss and Corbin, 1990). Core categories were then put into a matrix. Using Excel, data were tabulated and examined for frequencies of similar information.

RESULTS

As shown in Table 1, data from the entire sample indicated that themes perceived to be important for a good quality of life in different contexts included

TABLE 1. Recurrent QoL Issues Specific to Deaf and Hard of Hearing Individuals Reported by 49 Youths in Various Contexts

Home	School	Community
being able to communicate with family members	teachers understand and support the needs of deaf or hard of hearing youths	being able to participate in sports and other community activities
being comfortable with one's identity as deaf or hard of hearing	interpreters are proficient in sign language and sign clearly	having access to communication technology such as pagers and videophones
parents' ability to understand and communicate in sign language		work experience
feeling included in family conversations		having friends who are deaf or hearing

being comfortable with one's deaf or hard of hearing identity, having deaf and hearing friends, having access to communication technology such as pagers and videophones, being able to communicate with family members, and participating in sports or other community activities (Skalicky, Kushalnagar, Topolski, Schick, Edwards, & Patrick, 2010).

Although some individual differences surfaced, the deaf and hard of hearing Latino youth participants in this study were similar in that they included cultural values as an important aspect of a good quality of life for an individual who is deaf or hard of hearing and Latino. Recurrent themes that emerged as particular contributions to quality of life among these young people from Spanish-speaking families included communication access to social participation at large family gatherings; knowledge of Spanish; and family visits to Mexico (see Table 2).

TABLE 2. Selected Recurrent Issues Reported by 11 Latino Deaf and Hard of Hearing Youths from Spanish-Speaking Families

Communication Access	Language	Sociocultural Experience
perceived ability to participate in large family gatherings	perceived ability to understand Spanish	opportunities to visit home country (Mexico)
family and relatives who try different ways to communicate	perceived ability to speak Spanish	opportunities to venture outside neighborhoods; feeling of safety

Working within the theoretical framework of thematic analysis, the concepts were based on recurrent themes. Three main concepts (communication access, language, and sociocultural experience) appeared in all interviews with Latino deaf or hard of hearing youths from Spanish-speaking families. Although the research on how these young people perceived their quality of life has focused on home, school, and community, being the only nonfluent user of Spanish was clearly a communication barrier for these young people, whose Spanish-speaking families value large gatherings. Said one of the participants, "We keep trying. We never give up. My grandmother never gives up on what I want to say. I don't give up, either, because I want to learn. I myself, not them, get moody and frustrated because it is hard."

Because of the importance of their large family get-togethers, family members, especially parents and grandparents, tried their best to include the deaf and hard of hearing youths in these events. Despite this support, these young people commented that their quality of life would improve if they knew more Spanish and were able to communicate better on a one-to-one basis. As participants observed, "I want to learn Spanish, but I know only a little bit. It is awkward and hard." "I don't feel bad, but I get angry [at not being able to understand what Mother is saying]. So when I do that, I just, like, read a Spanish book, and I learn." "Well, most of the time I'm jealous because they [the participant's parents] . . . talk Spanish and communicate with other people that talk other languages, and I didn't try to learn fluent Spanish and communicate with them a little bit, and every time I try to say a word in Spanish, I say it wrong, and they think I'm trying to say a different word."

Interestingly, only one youth out of 11 participants asserted that his parents should learn American Sign Language to communicate with him. A possible explanation for the tendency of Latino deaf and hard of hearing youths to favor learning Spanish (over saying that the parents should also learn American Sign Language) is the cultural emphasis on the respect that young people are expected to show their parents.

Another commonality among these Latino deaf and hard of hearing youths was a positive outlook on home visits to Mexico, which is associated with a perceived better quality of life. These youths reported feeling happy when they were with their cousins or neighbors in their home country, where communication was described as better and more inclusive even when only gestures and broken vocabularies were used. It should be noted that these comments came primarily from those whose families immigrated to the United States when they were younger.

Quality of life is considered by some researchers to be affected by health-related conditions (Cella, 1995; Patrick & Erickson, 1988; Schipper, Clinch, & Olweny, 1996; Guyatt, Feeny, & Patrick, 1993), but in this study contextual factors such as communication access and language use were shown to be pertinent to perceived quality of life in young people who are deaf or hard of hearing regardless of their ethnic and cultural background.

CONCLUSION

The deaf or hard of hearing youth from Spanish-speaking families perceived ability to participate in family gatherings, Spanish knowledge, and family visits to Mexico as most pertinent to positive quality of life. These observations suggest that focus should be on helping these youth and their parents develop effective communication strategies that will result in improved parent-youth relationship and youth perceived quality of life. These combined with the youth's opportunity to participate in community and family activities (e.g. sports; travel to Mexico) can potentially ameliorate the negative effect associated with reduced communication access, low-income, and parent education status.

In a cross-sectional study of 231 deaf and hard of hearing young people in the United States, the youth's perceived ability to understand what parents say was strongly associated with perceived quality of life and reported depressive symptomatology (Kushalnagar et al., 2011), with poorer perceived quality of life and level of parent communication being associated with greater number of reported depressive symptoms. More recently, logistic regression analysis of 143 late adolescents and young adults who were no longer living at home indicated that those who retrospectively reported being able to understand some to none of what their parents said were at least 6.6 times more likely to report current depressive symptomatology than others who retrospectively reported being able to understand most or all of what their parents said (Kushalnagar, Bruce, Sutton, & Leigh, 2015). Cumulative impacts on later mental health outcomes can result from the combination of youth perceived ability to understand home communication and youth perceived quality of life. This can potentially outweigh factors in the school that predict the youth's motivation and ability to succeed in school. A large body of literature consistently suggest that parental involvement and communication with the youth has a positive impact on the youth's academic achievement and psychological adjustment, even after controlling for other factors that are associated with the outcomes (Desforges & Abouchaar, 2003; Karbach et al., 2013; Wang & Sheikh-Khalil, 2014).

This qualitative study is limited by the small sample size and the origin of deaf and hard of hearing Latino youth's families that speak Spanish. All participants' families are from Mexico, and most reside in the Southwest region of USA. Their experiences may not be representative of broader populations that include deaf and hard of hearing Latino youth from non-Mexican, Spanish-speaking families. By expanding the focus of this study to multiple regions or countries (e.g., Dominican Republic, Puerto Rico, Cuba) additional data can be obtained to substantiate or expand the findings from the present study. The absence of literature regarding the issue of bidirectional-bilingual communication (fluency in both American Sign Language and home language by both deaf or hard of hearing youth and their parents) also became apparent during this study. With the changing population of deaf and hard of hearing youths in the United States, the potential influence of bidirectional-bilingual communication must be integrated into YQoL models for young people who are deaf or hard of hearing and analyzed as a potential barrier.

Parental involvement, family communication, cultural background and socioeconomic status influence how Latino deaf and hard of hearing youth view their parents' contribution to their quality of life and how they interact with peers who are similar or different from them. By understanding how the Latino deaf and hard of hearing youth perceive the impacts of language differences on their quality of life, psychology and healthcare providers, as well as school personnel, will be able to work more effectively with all youths as well as parents of children to improve and maintain positive quality of life in general.

REFERENCES

Addy, S., Engelhardt, W., & Skinner, C. (2013). *Basic facts about low-income children, 2011: Children under age 18.* New York: National Center for Children in Poverty, Columbia University, Mailman School of Public Health.

Blumer, H. (1969). *Symbolic interactionism: Perspective and method.* Englewood Cliffs, NJ: Prentice-Hall.

Bronfenbrenner, U. (1979). *The ecology of human development.* Cambridge, MA: Harvard University Press.

Cella, D. (1995). Measuring quality of life in palliative care. *Seminars in Oncology, 22,* 73–81.

Christensen, K., & Delgado, G. (1993). *Multicultural issues in deafness.* White Plains, NY: Longman.

Delgado, G. (2001). *Hispanic/Latino deaf students in our schools.* Research report. Knoxville: Postsecondary Education Consortium, University of Tennessee.

Desforges, C., & Abouchaar, A. (2003). *The impact of parental involvement, parental support and family education on pupil achievement and adjustment: A review of literature.* London: DfES Publications.

Edwards, T. C., Huebner, C. E., Connell, F. A., & Patrick, D. L. (2002). Adolescent quality of life, part I: conceptual and measurement model. *Journal of Adolescence, 25,* 275–286.

Glaser, B. G., & Strauss, A. L. (1967). *Discovery of grounded theory: Strategies for qualitative research.* Chicago: Aldine.

Guyatt, G. H., Feeny, D. H., & Patrick, D. L. (1993). Measuring health-related quality of life. *Annals of Internal Medicine, 118,* 622–628.

Karbach, J., Gottschling, J., Spengler, M., Hegewald, K., & Spinath, F. M. (2013). Parental involvement and general cognitive ability as predictors of domain-specific academic achievement in early adolescence. *Learning and Instruction, 23,* 43–51.

Kushalnagar, P., Topolski, T. D., Schick, B., Edwards, T. E., Skalicky, A. M., & Patrick, D. L. (2011). Mode of communication: Perceived level of understanding and perceived quality of life in youth who are deaf or hard-of-hearing. *Journal of Deaf Studies and Deaf Education, 16,* 512–523.

Kushalnagar, P., Bruce, S., Sutton, T., & Leigh, I. W. (2015). *Early communicative stress is gender-specific and linked to adulthood depression.* Poster presented at the annual meeting of the American Psychological Association, Toronto, Canada.

Patrick, D. P., Edwards, T. C., Skalicky, A. M., Leng, M., Topolski, T., Schick, B., Kushalnagar, P., & Sie, K. (2011). Measurement properties of a quality of life instrument for youth who are deaf or hard-of-hearing (YQOL-DHH). *Archives of Otolaryngology: Head & Neck Surgery.* PMID: 21493349.

Patrick, D. L., & Erickson, P. (1988). Assessing health-related quality of life for clinical decision making. In S. R. Walker & R. M. Rosser (Eds.), *Quality of life: Assessment and application* (p. 22). Lancaster, UK: MTP Press.

Patrick, D. L., Edwards, T. C., & Topolski, T. D. (2002) Adolescent quality of life, part II: initial validation of a new instrument. *Journal of Adolescence, 25*, 287–300.

Schipper, H., Clinch, J. J., & Olweny, C. L. M. (1996). Quality of life studies: Definitions and conceptual issues. In B. Spilker (Ed.), *Quality of life and pharmacoeconomics in clinical trials* (pp. 11–23). Philadelphia: Lippincott-Raven.

Skalicky, A. M., Topolski, T. D., Schick, B., Edwards, T. C., & Patrick, D. L. (2010). *Perception of quality of life among youth who are deaf or hard-of-hearing.* Poster session at the conference of the International Society of Quality of Life Research, London.

Strauss, A., & Corbin, J. (1990). *Basics of qualitative research: Techniques and procedures for developing grounded theory.* Newbury Park, CA: Sage.

US Census Bureau. (2011). *The Hispanic population in the United States: 2011.* Retrieved March 22, 2013, from http://www.census.gov/population/hispanic/data/2011.html

Wang, M. T., & Sheikh-Khalil, S. (2014). Does parental involvement matter for student achievement and mental health in high school? *Child Development, 85*(2), 610–625.

Part 3

Deaf Children and Their Families

10

Mental Health Problems in Deaf Children and Adolescents: Part I—Epidemiology, Etiology, and Cultural, Linguistic, and Developmental Aspects

Tiejo van Gent

Being deaf in a world oriented to the needs of hearing people increases a child's vulnerability to mental health problems. Understanding why this is and how it happens helps explain both normal development and psychopathology (Hindley & van Gent, 2002). Of all deaf children, 90–95% are born into hearing families; thus the views of their parents is very important. One of the major challenges faced by deaf children (i.e., children with bilateral, severe-to-profound hearing impairment) is obtaining access to meaningful communication through a visuospatial signed and/or spoken language. Health professionals have to take into account the fact that many deaf people do not view themselves as having an impairment or a handicap but rather as having their own language and culture. In this chapter "deaf" children refers to those with permanent, bilateral, severe-to-profound hearing impairment. In addition, we briefly discuss the effects of otitis media with

Author's note: This chapter and the following chapter are updated and extended versions of T. van Gent, (2012), Mental health problems in deaf children and adolescents. In T. van Gent, *Mental health problems in deaf and severely hard of hearing children and adolescents. Findings on prevalence, pathogenesis and clinical complexities, and implications for prevention, diagnosis and intervention* (pp. 23–80), PhD thesis, Leiden University, Netherlands. The dissertation itself concerns a broadly renewed and adapted revision of P. A. Hindley & T. van Gent, (2002), Psychiatric aspects of specific hearing impairments, in M. Rutter & E. Taylor (Eds.), *Child and adolescent psychiatry* (4th ed.) (pp. 842–857). Oxford: Blackwell Science.

effusion (OME), as well as the mental health of hearing children of deaf parents and of children with a combination of a hearing and a visual impairment (i.e., deaf-blindness).

EPIDEMIOLOGY OF DEAFNESS

A bilateral hearing impairment (HI) is usually described quantitatively in terms of the unaided, averaged, pure-tone decibel (dB) hearing threshold for noise in the better hearing ear. Degrees of impairment may be categorized as mild, moderate, severe, and profound, but parameters for decibel thresholds may vary. For example, Stephens (2001) defines mild impairment as 20–40 dB, moderate as 41–70 dB, severe as 71–95, and profound as ≥ 96 dB, whereas Walch, Anderhuber, Köle, and Berghold (2000) describe mild as 15–30 dB, moderate as 31–60 dB, severe as 61–90 dB, and profound as ≥ 91 dB. In European countries, more than 1 in 1,000 children are likely to have permanent, bilateral congenital HI of moderate or greater severity (Davis & Parving, 1994; Fortnum & Davis, 1997). The prevalence of HI rises to 50–90% among children 9 years of age and older (Fortnum, Summerfield, Marshall, Davis, & Bamford, 2001). The postnatal rise in the prevalence of HI can be explained by genetic progressive HI and, to a lesser extent, by acquired HI (approximately 4–9% of overall prevalence) or delayed confirmation of congenital HI (Fortnum et al., 2001). The prevalence of HI has not changed over time (De Graaf, Knippers, & Bijl, 1997; Fortnum et al., 2001). A systematic review of population-based studies in developed countries on reported distributions of causes of permanent bilateral childhood HI in children with a loss of ≥ 40 dB (Korver et al., 2011) shows weighted means of 30.4% for HI of hereditary origin (syndromic and nonsyndromic), 19.2% for pre-, peri-, or postnatally acquired HI, and 48.3% for unknown causes. However, over time the relative distribution of etiologies changes. Findings from a large population study in the UK suggests that cases of syndromic and perinatal origin (including severe prematurity) have increased, and HI of unknown, prenatal (e.g., rubella) and postnatal (e.g., meningitis) etiologies have decreased (Fortnum et al., 2002). Reported rates of etiologies vary across the included categories of hearing level and also with the inclusion of unknown etiologies (ibid.). It is highly likely that technological improvements in diagnosis will reduce the number of cases of unknown etiology in favor of cases with known origins, including recessive hereditary causes, single gene mutations, subclinical viral infections (e.g., cytomegalovirus), and inner-ear malformations (Walch et al., 2000).

Nine out of 10 cases of hearing impairment are sensorineural, most commonly related to sensory dysfunction in the inner ear. Less often, the hearing loss involves the eighth nerve, the vestibulocochlear nerve, or more central auditory pathways in the central nervous system. The most common cause of a peripheral conductive hearing loss (i.e., a loss caused by a defect in the middle or external ear) is otitis media, which may physically impede the conduction of sound. Acute otitis media (OM) is probably the most common reason for consultation with general practitioners in the preschool years (Haggard & Hughes, 1991). Although OM does not usually cause permanent HI, otitis media with effusion (OME) can lead to fluctuating HI, which affects approximately 10–30% children 2–7 years of age (ibid.).

In addition, HI may be further classified as nonsyndromic and syndromic. About 70% of hereditary HI is considered nonsyndromic as it is not accompanied by other clinical symptoms, whereas the remaining 30% is considered syndromic as it is combined with abnormalities, malformations, or dysfunctions in one or more organ systems (Walch et al., 2000). An important example of syndromic autosomal recessive HI is Usher syndrome, with the co-occurrence of sensorineural deafness and a gradual loss of vision due to retinitis pigmentosa (RP). Another example is the Jervell and Lange-Nielsen syndrome, with combined sensorineural HI and prolonged QT interval leading to arrhythmias and possibly dangerous, syncopal episodes. Examples of autosomal dominant syndromes are Waardenburg syndrome, with sensorineural HI, pigmentation abnormalities of the eyes (heterochromia of the iris), hair (usually a patch of white hair), and skin, and dystopia canthorum (wide space between the inner corners of the eyes), and branchio-oto-renal syndrome, combining conductive, sensorineural, or mixed HI with ear malformations, branchial fistulae, and cysts, and renal malformations (Gorlin, Toriello, & Cohen, 1995). Congenital rubella syndrome, the co-occurrence of profound HI with impairments in other organ systems such as the heart (congenital heart defects), the eyes (e.g., cataracts, retinopathy), and the brain (e.g., mental retardation, movement and coordination problems, microcephaly) is an example of nongenetic syndromic HI (ibid.). Other examples are very low birth weight and meningitis, both of which may be accompanied by brain abnormalities. Universal neonatal hearing screening is crucial for early detection of additional impairments.

CULTURAL ASPECTS

Though many, particularly hearing, people perceive deafness and hearing loss primarily as a disability, an impairment, and/or a physical disorder, deaf people are socioculturally and linguistically heterogeneous. For many deaf people, being deaf means being part of a unique culture with its own language, traditions, and values (Maxwell-McCaw & Zea, 2011). In addition, one sociocultural view of deafness suggests that Deaf culture has three main characteristics: a primarily visual experience of the world; membership in a sociocultural minority; and the use of sign language (Meadow-Orlans & Erting, 2000). With a large majority of deaf children having hearing parents, membership in the Deaf community is acquired mainly outside the family. The community contains only few native speakers as only 5–10% of deaf children are born to one or both deaf parents (Quigley & Paul,

1984; Singleton & Tittle, 2000). To varying degrees, deaf people, as well as their hearing family members, may identify with the Deaf community, with both the Deaf and the hearing communities, or predominantly with the majority culture of the hearing community (Hintermair, 2007; Maxwell-McCaw & Zea, 2011). Another subgroup may lack a clear preference for any of these acculturation styles (Hintermair, 2007). At present at least four factors influence the process of identity formation. First, the educational status of native sign languages has progressed in the last 20 years with the development of bilingual/bicultural educational programs. In many developed countries, education has become more inclusive, aiming at more social integration and better academic involvement for all (Marschark, 2007). Third, the development of hearing screening programs for newborn children has greatly contributed to the earlier identification of hearing loss and the establishment of early intervention programs that focus on family support and communication. Finally, the introduction of the cochlear implant (CI), an electronic device that delivers hearing sensations by electrically stimulating the auditory nerve of the inner ear, has provided many children with more access to the world of sound and spoken language. In summary, deaf children may benefit from these and other developments as long as their strengths and special needs (discussed) are sufficiently addressed.

SIGN LANGUAGE

Sign languages develop naturally wherever groups of deaf people come together (Groce & Whiting, 1988) and are independent of the dominant spoken languages. For example, British Sign Language (BSL) and American Sign Language (ASL) have less in common at a lexical level than do ASL and French Sign Language, inasmuch as ASL is historically influenced by the Langue des Signes Française (LSF) (Armstrong & Wilcox, 2003). Moreover, all sign languages have in common the expression of semantic and grammatical concepts by movements of the hands, the face, and the upper body (Hindley & van Gent, 2002). They differ from spoken languages in that they are visuospatially organized languages in which meaning can be transferred simultaneously by the hands, face (i.e., eye gaze and facial expression), and body movements in the visual sign space, in contrast to the more sequential transfer of meaning in words in spoken languages. Most signed sentence structures follow a topic-comment format in contrast to the subject-object-verb structure of most spoken languages (Sutton-Spence & Woll, 1999). Typically, sign languages use spatial descriptors to map spatial relations topographically (using many classifier signs, which can refer to subjects and other nouns), as well as non-topographic sentences, which use fewer classifiers (MacSweeney et al., 2002).

    The study of sign language adds to our understanding of the ontology of language (Stokoe, 1998) and of the neural processes underpinning language function

(Corina, 1999). Evidence suggests that language preference in early infancy is not speech specific (Krentz & Corina, 2008) and that hearing and deaf children are equally predisposed to attend to linguistic and prosodic features of motherese in speech or sign (Masataka, 2003). In their first year of life, infants specialize in processing either visual or auditory linguistic signals as their native language, while their abilities in distinguishing the other (i.e., nonnative, linguistic signals) decline at the end of the first year (Baker, Michnick Golinkoff, & Petitto 2006; Krentz & Corina, 2008). Neural systems underlying signed and spoken language processing show many similarities. Both make special use of the left perisylvian regions of the brain. This specialization, which reflects the visuospatial or auditory input modalities for signed and spoken language (Campbell, MacSweeney, & Waters, 2008), is most likely determined by the demands of the perceptual task of visuospatial or auditory language processing (e.g., "compositionality, syntax, and the requirements of mapping coherent concepts onto a communicable form") rather than by the acoustic or articulatory prerequisites for hearing or speaking (ibid., p. 17). Other studies also suggest right hemisphere involvement in signed languages, but whether this reflects visuospatial modality- or nonmodality-specific functions; extragrammatical, prosodic, or topic coherence functions; or still other conditions remains to be elucidated (Rönnberg, Söderfeldt, & Risberg, 2000; Campbell et al., 2008).

DEAF CHILDREN AND DEAF PARENTS

The language development of deaf children of deaf parents is comparable to that of hearing children (Petitto & Marentette, 1991; Caselli & Volterra, 1989). Deaf parents may have greater sensitivity to the early communicative efforts of their infants than do hearing parents of deaf infants (Smith-Gray & Koester, 1995). They may be more likely to perceive their deaf infants' bodily signals as attempts to communicate, and so they reciprocate. They may use a variety of methods to gain their infants' attention (Harris, 2001) and to create joint attention (Loots & Devisé, 2003). Deaf mothers are more consistent in signing in the child's signing space, using visual (moving hands) or tactile signals (touching physically) to attract visual attention, and waiting to obtain the child's visual attention before signing (ibid.). They adapt their signing in ways that may be considered parallel to hearing parents' spoken "motherese" (Erting, Prezioso, & O'Grady Hynes, 1989; Masataka, 1996). Visual and communicative attunement may promote a child's development in many ways. For instance, early signers have been found to be more proficient than late signers in learning spoken language (Mayberry, Lock, & Kazmi, 2002). Moreover, visuotactile communication, especially sign language, facilitates intersubjectivity (i.e., the exchange and sharing of both linguistic and symbolic meaning between parents–deaf child pairs) (Loots, Devisé, & Jacquet, 2005). In addition, exposure to a visual language and culture may promote the development of visual engagement, executive functions such as attention regulation, inhibitory control, and self-monitoring, and sociocognitive skills such as theory of mind; (discussed later) (Corina & Singleton, 2009).

DEAF CHILDREN AND HEARING PARENTS

The vast majority (90–95%) of parents of deaf children are hearing. Most of them will have had no prior contact with deaf people and may experience considerable emotional distress when they realize their child is deaf (Freeman, Malkin, & Hastings, 1975). Moreover, each parent may respond differently, in terms of anxiousness and feelings of guilt, to the child's deafness (Meadow-Orlans, 1995; Marschark, 2007). From a cultural perspective on deafness, it is important that parents learn to recognize that their child is different and does not necessarily have a disability (Young, 1999). The family's response to the consequences of a child's deafness in general reflects their coping skills, social network (Danek, 1988), cultural backgrounds, and belief systems. Many parents come to embrace a cultural construction of deafness, but many struggle with the notion of it as much as with disability (Hindley, 1999). In general, parents who receive adequate social and emotional support (Calderon & Greenberg, 1999) may be very capable of coping with the demands of having a deaf child (Marschark, 2007) and do not necessarily exhibit more stress than hearing parents of hearing children (Pipp-Siegel, Sedey, & Yoshinaga-Itano, 2002). In other cases, the experience of having a deaf child may be difficult to cope with if hearing parents regard hearing and speaking as innate, core aspects of themselves and consequently of their expectations of their child and their interaction with him or her (Erting, 1982). A number of risk factors for high stress among parents are lower income, lower perceived support, serious daily problems, the presence of disabilities in addition to hearing loss, serious language delay, and less severe hearing loss (Pipp-Siegel et al., 2002). The hidden handicap of a milder hearing loss and profitable residual hearing in a hearing environment may make it more difficult to estimate the impact of the loss on the child's functioning and to recognize his or her special needs (ibid.), as is also the case with children who have other hidden and relative disabilities (Miyahara & Piek, 2006).

Hearing mothers of deaf infants have been found to be less responsive to their children than either deaf mothers of deaf infants or hearing mothers of hearing infants (Spencer & Meadow-Orlans, 1996). This diminished responsiveness may stem from a lesser sensitivity to the deaf infants' visual signals (Spencer, Bodner-Johnson, & Gutfreund, 1992; Prendergast & McCollum, 1996; Harris, 2000) and is likely to have implications for the child's development in all domains (Hindley & van Gent, 2002). Many hearing parents have also been found to be more directive and controlling in their interactions with their deaf children when compared with hearing-hearing dyads and with deaf-deaf dyads (Marschark, 1993). This may derive from difficulties in managing divided attention (Harris, 2000) but may also be a response to the children's delayed language development. Programs for neonatal hearing screening and early intervention have greatly contributed to the provision of early social support for and information to hearing parents, thus creating many more possibilities for parents to find effective assistance in adapting to the needs of their deaf child. They have also helped promote effective communication between hearing parents and their deaf children. Such programs have focused on both visual and spoken language, as well as social-emotional development (Moeller, 2000; Sass-Lehrer & Bodner-Johnson, 2003; Yoshinaga-Itano, 2003). It is important to note here that, in addition to the age of detection and early enrollment, parental involvement (including emotional availability and effective communicative interaction) has been found to be a powerful predictor of language development (Moeller, 2000; Yoshinaga-Itano, 2003), and this association may be even stronger for deaf children than for their hearing peers (Pressman, Pipp-Siegel, Yoshinaga-Itano, Kubicek, & Emde, 2000).

LANGUAGE DEVELOPMENT IN DEAF CHILDREN

Infants have an innate capacity to learn any language regardless of modality (Baker et al., 2006; Marschark, 2007). The onset of babbling marks one of the earliest stages of linguistic development (Schick, 2003). Babbling with the hands, a rhythmic, syllabically organized linguistic activity with the hands, has been observed in both deaf and hearing very young infants who learn sign language from birth (Baker et al., 2006; Petitto et al., 1991; Petitto et al., 2004), and has also been demonstrated in hearing infants without prior exposure to signing (Baker et al., 2006). In deaf children, vocal babbling decreases during the first year of life, unlike in hearing children (Marschark, 2007). In general, a gradual decline in the capacity to discriminate between and produce language elements (phonetic units) in the least familiar (i.e., least practiced, nonnative language) has been observed in both deaf and hearing infants by the end of the first year of life (Baker et al., 2006; Krentz & Corina, 2008). Taking into account a considerable variation in children, deaf children of deaf parents produce sign language at about the same mean age as hearing children of hearing parents produce spoken language (Marschark, 2007), but the communicative circumstances are less favorable for the majority of deaf children (i.e., deaf children of hearing parents). Hearing parents use two features of language with their deaf child (Marschark, 1993). First, they tend to simplify both their spoken and signed language and, in the case of sign language, drop important function signs. Second, interactions between deaf children and hearing parents tend to be shorter and less complex and contain fewer questions and self-references. As a result, communication is frequently impoverished, and deaf children of hearing parents may refer more frequently to concrete themes and less to more abstract concepts as a reflection of these patterns of communication with their parents (Marschark, 2007).

Moreover, many hearing parents experience considerable difficulties in acquiring fluent signing skills and gain only limited proficiency in sign language. Much the same applies to hearing teachers of deaf children (Wood, Wood, Griffiths, & Howarth 1986; Power, Wood, & Wood, 1990). They tend to be more controlling, use more conversational repair strategies, and initiate fewer interactions. This controlling style is often associated with both fewer questions and less elaborate answers from pupils. In fact, compared with their hearing peers, deaf children who are subject to more restricted communication discourse patterns with hearing parents and teachers (Hauser, Lukomski, & Hillman, 2008) are at risk of experiencing less diversity (Marschark, 2007), less incidental learning (Calderon & Greenberg, 2003), and less exposure to a variety of cause-effect relationships reflecting differences in problem solving and a tendency to focus on individual item processing rather than on sequential processing and relationships among items (Marschark, 2003, 2007). Notwithstanding advances in visual spatial processing, deaf children may be less likely to focus on sequential processing and relations among concepts and more on individual items (ibid.; Marschark & Wauters, 2008).

Early and later sign language learning does not impede but instead tends to favor the learning of spoken and written English (Spencer, Gantz, & Knutson, 2004; Yoshinaga-Itano, 2006). Studies with hearing bilinguals, whose languages are both spoken, show that bilingualism promotes the development of executive control functions such as attention, planning, and categorization (Baker, 2007; Bialystok & Craik, 2010; Bialystok, 2011) and outweighs the disadvantages, such as smaller vocabularies and less rapid access to lexical items (Bialystok & Craik, 2010). However, the beneficial effects of bilingualism may be somewhat different for deaf bilingual children than for hearing bilingual children as sign languages are not equivalent to spoken languages (Knoors & Marschark, 2012).

Delayed linguistic input affects language acquisition, and with increasing ages of exposure a gradual decline in average proficiency occurs (Newport, Bavelier, & Neville, 2001). When deaf children are exposed to gestures but not to formal signing, they tend to develop their own gestural systems, often called "home signs" (Hindley & van Gent, 2002). Home signs contain many properties of natural languages and appear to convey a second-language learning advantage when formal sign language is encountered later in life (Morford, 1998). Even a new sign language may develop through interaction between previously isolated adult home signers and young deaf children exposed to the gestural system in a new deaf community, as has been shown to happen in Nicaragua (Goldin-Meadow, 2010; Kegl, Senghas, & Coppola, 1999; Senghas, 2010). When deaf children are presented with signed versions of spoken language, their expressive signing increasingly approximates native sign language, particularly in the use of spatial grammatical principles (Supalla, 1991). When deaf children of hearing parents receive good-quality sign input, their sign language development parallels spoken language development in hearing children in sequence but not always in rate (Marschark, 1993).

Earlier neonatal hearing screening identification (below 6 months) and early intervention programs are associated with better receptive and expressive spoken language development in deaf infants (Yoshinaga-Itano & Apuzzo, 1998; Sass-Lehrer & Bodner-Johnson, 2003). The use of cochlear implants (CI) with younger children has raised parents' expectations with regard to their children's potential to develop spoken language and has been shown to lead to significant gains in language development (Meyer, Svirsky, Kirk, & Miyamoto, 1998). After initial opposition, many Deaf communities now support the use of CIs as a communicative alternative for deaf children (Christiansen & Leigh, 2004). Cochlear implants do not change deaf children into hearing children (Marschark, 2007), and children and adolescents who have implants remain at a disadvantage in acquiring spoken language and academic skills when compared to hearing peers. Even with a functioning implant, most of them will still experience moderate to severe hearing loss with estimated improvements of nearly 30dB (Blamey et al., 2001) and will still rely on more limited information than do hearing children. Second, many already experienced a delay in spoken language development before the implant and thus lack an understanding of the structure of information (Marschark, 2007). Third, part of the auditory information will be missed when the implant malfunctions or background noise interferes (Knoors & Marschark, 2012). Although language development shows more progression in children with implants than in those with conventional hearing aids, a CI still rarely corrects for delays prior to implantation (Bat-Chava, Martin, & Kosciw, 2004). Studies show advantages in speech perception and production, reading abilities, and academic achievement (Beadle et al., 2005; Spencer & Marschark, 2003) for children with CIs. Other variables have been reported to have beneficial effects on speech and language performance of children with implants. Examples include degree, age of onset and etiology of hearing impairment, age at implantation (the younger, the better), the length of CI experience, increased involvement in spoken language before and after the operation, total daily time of CI use, nonverbal intelligence (Wie, Falkenberg, Tvete, & Tomblin, 2007), pre- and postoperative sign language experience (Connor, Hieber, Arts, & Zwolan, 2000; Yoshinaga-Itano, 2006), quality of parental guidance and professional therapy following implantation, the child's cognitive abilities, the quality of parent-child communication, parental hearing status, and the child's temperament (Marschark, 2007). Some early intervention programs provide mentorship from a deaf person, whose support with respect to communication and to cultural awareness of deafness seems to foster the children's language development (Watkins, Pitman, & Walden, 1998; Young, 1999).

COGNITIVE DEVELOPMENT

Since the 1950s an increasing awareness of the effects of language on cognitive development has led to the formulation of specific nonverbal intelligence tests (e.g., Snijders Oomen; Leiter; Hiskey Nebraska; see Blennerhasset, 2000) for deaf children and to the standardization of performance scales in other instruments, such as the Wechsler Intelligence Scale for Children.

Comparable performance IQ scores for deaf and hearing peers have been reported (Maller, 2003; Mayberry, 2002; Vernon, 1968/2005), but verbal IQs for the former tend to be one standard deviation below the mean for the latter (Maller, 2003). With deaf people, verbal IQs may be used as a measure of literacy skills and academic achievement rather than as a measure of intelligence (Blennerhasset, 2000). Nevertheless, even on nonverbal tests, deaf children have been shown to score below the level of their hearing peers (Braden, 1994; Marschark, 1993). Such apparent discrepancies might be explained by factors related to the tests in use (e.g., not being truly independent of language or culture) and/or the heterogeneity of the deaf population under study. Lower performance by deaf children of hearing parents may be explained by late or incomplete spoken and/or sign language exposure, resulting in poor development of mental language representations and working memory (Mayberry, 2002). High performance IQ scores in children with (nonsyndromal) hereditary deafness (Kusché, Greenberg, & Garfield, 1983) and children with signing deaf parents (Sisco & Anderson, 1980; Zwiebel, 1987) can be explained by the ideas that intelligence may be partly inherited. Early language exposure may facilitate intelligence (Vernon, 1968/2005), deaf parents may be better prepared to meet a deaf child's early learning needs (Sisco & Anderson, 1980), or learning a visuospatial language may stimulate that child's visuospatial abilities (Bellugi et al., 1990).

Possible risks for impaired cognitive development in some deaf children include central nervous system damage; lack of communication; limited social interaction; overcontrol by caregivers; restriction of experiences as a consequence of language deprivation and restricted incidental learning; and lack of exposure to sound (Marschark, 1993), which affects the ability to integrate distal and proximal events (Campbell, 1998).

Studies have shown both similarities and differences in the cognitive functioning of deaf and hearing individuals. For instance, deaf children may lag behind hearing children in their development of conversation or may show shorter memory spans perhaps because of less efficient retrieval strategies, lesser reliance on relations among concepts, or lower strength in associative connections (Marschark, 2003). Generally, deaf children show less verbal creativity when assessed through tests using spoken rather than sign language (Marschark, 2007). Deaf children rely more than hearing children on visual-perceptual thinking and visual memory and less on abstract thinking. On the other hand, deaf individuals who use sign language tend to have an advantage over nonsigning hearing and deaf people in visuospatial processing and learning. For instance, native signers are better at distinguishing facial features related to sign language information (Bettger, Emmorey, McCullough, & Bellugi, 1997; McCullough & Emmorey, 1997). All signers are better than nonsigners in generating mental images on the basis of information in long-term memory. They are better at manipulating them visually in physical space (i.e., using space to encode spatial information), especially by shifting reference and perspective of referents during discourse, and at the exact representation of visuospatial relations within scenes (Emmorey, Kosslyn, & Bellugi, 1993; Emmorey & Kosslyn, 1996; Talbot & Haude, 1993). Moreover, native signers, both deaf and hearing, are more aware of movement (Neville & Lawson, 1987) in the visual periphery than other nonsigning individuals, but this might be more the result of early auditory deprivation than language modality (Proksch & Bavelier, 2002). The impact of such visuospatial, memory, and attentional differences on daily problem solving and learning is complex and warrants further study (Rönnberg et al., 2000; Marschark, 2007).

ACADEMIC ACHIEVEMENT IN DEAF CHILDREN

Even when deaf children and their hearing peers are found to show comparable nonverbal IQ scores, some cognitive skills and knowledge are transferred through language, and better language is associated with better cognitive and school-related academic performance. This may put deaf children at a disadvantage, and many do show significant underachievement in reading, writing, and mathematical concepts (Stinson & Kluwin, 2003; Traxler, 2000); of these, reading is probably the most difficult skill for many students (Antia, Jones, Reed, & Kreimeyer, 2009). For about 50% of 18-year-old deaf and hard of hearing adolescents, reading skills are equivalent to those of hearing 9-year-old children, compared to 1% of their hearing peers (Traxler, 2000). It is probably relevant that most (prelingual) deaf children learn to read and write in what is effectively a second language. Some deaf children have no basic problem with phonological coding but have a limited vocabulary and a restricted knowledge of syntax. Differences in the amount and organization of knowledge in semantic memory (Marschark, 2003) and diminished experience of the interaction among the semantic, syntactic, and pragmatic components of spoken language (Campbell, 1998) may be influential.

Strategies to improve deaf children's reading and writing abilities include accessing reading through sign language (Prinz & Strong, 1998; Hoffmeister, de Villiers, Engen, & Topol, 1997) and offering spoken language by presenting phonological code in the form of handshapes held alongside the face as in cued speech (Campbell, 1998). In addition, detailed knowledge of sign language syntax enhances children's metalinguistic skills, enabling them to decode English

(Hoffmeister et al., 1997). However, many deaf children need further bridging skills (Prinz & Strong, 1998), such as enhancing recognition of phonological code (Campbell, 1998) and recognizing letter-word patterns through the use of finger-spelling and sign initialization (Padden & Ramsey, 1998). Probably the best outcomes for literacy in deaf children occur when children are exposed at an early age to either fluent signed or spoken language in general (Mayberry, 2002), as well as to the language they will learn to read (Marschark, 2007).

As a result of earlier educational experiences at home and school, many deaf children and adolescents demonstrate a cognitive style characterized by an example-bound or instrumentally dependent approach to the environment (ibid.). The tendency to focus on individual items rather than on relationships between or among them may affect performance in a variety of domains such as reading, recalling, and interpreting content and recognizing relational information. Deaf children may be especially at risk of underachieving in settings that are primarily hearing oriented and relatively unfamiliar with differences in cognitive styles and learning strategies used by deaf children and young people (Marschark & Wauters, 2008; Hauser & Marschark, 2008). Thus, educational intervention could beneficially find ways to enhance reflective problem solving, help deaf children become more aware of and involved in their own learning (Marschark, 2007), mobilize support, and promote validation of personal competencies (Calderon & Greenberg, 1993; Marschark, 2007; van Gent, Goedhart, Knoors, Westenberg, & Treffers, 2012). Longitudinal research suggests that cochlear implantation has important long-term benefits for social participation, academic achievement, and later employment (Beadle et al., 2005). However, since early cochlear implantation reduces but does not eliminate lags in literacy, children with implants still need as much support as other hard of hearing children (Marschark, 2007). Further research is warranted into how such effects compare to long-term outcomes for unaided young people or young people with hearing aids in educational settings with appropriate academic and social support services.

SOCIAL AND EMOTIONAL DEVELOPMENT

Deaf infants show the same range of emotional states as hearing infants (Snitzer, Reilly, McIntire, & Bellugi, 1989) but tend to develop smaller emotional vocabularies and be less competent at recognizing other people's emotional states (Greenberg & Kusché, 1993). For a number of deaf children, the inability to articulate experience linguistically and to label emotional states may be one of the factors leading to gaps in social-emotional development (Calderon & Greenberg, 2003). However, the impact of deafness is influenced by various factors such as quality of family environment, parental adaptation to deafness, the nature of school and community resources, the child's personal characteristics, and the child's interactions with the surrounding environment (ibid.).

Deaf children of hearing mothers have been shown to exhibit less social initiative, less compliance, creativity, and enjoyment in their interactions with their mothers and more behavioral problems than their hearing peers (Lederberg & Mobley, 1990), while deaf children of deaf parents have been shown to display less impulsive and more reflective cognitive styles than deaf children of hearing parents (Harris, 1978). These types of differences, found also in older studies, may be the consequence of communicative and social deprivation and distorted parent-child interaction (Feinstein, 1983), which may diminish with improved communication between parents and child (Sinkkonen, 1994). Reduced communication, miscommunications, and difficulties in gaining and sustaining visual attention with a deaf child due to a lack of communicative skills or to communicative insecurity on the part of hearing caregivers may hamper opportunities to develop shared meaning and interactional reciprocity (Koester, 1994; Steinberg, 2000; Traci & Koester, 2003).

The preschool friendship patterns of deaf and hearing children do not differ, but deaf preschool children are more likely to use visual communication with their deaf peers than with their hearing peers (Lederberg, Ryan, & Robbins, 1986). Studies that examine the social-emotional functioning of students with a hearing impairment in different school settings have yielded mixed results. Although attending mainstream schools has been associated with the experience of loneliness, social rejection, and low global self-esteem among deaf students (Farrugia & Austin, 1980, more recent studies have found no relation between the type of school setting and loneliness (Kluwin, 1999) or global self-esteem (van Gurp, 2001; Kluwin, Stinson, & Colarossi, 2002). Multidimensional self-concept studies suggest that populations of deaf children or adolescents may show low self-perceived competence in the social domains only (Capelli, Daniels, Durieux-Smith, McGrath, & Neuss, 1995; van Gent et al., 2012). Low global self-esteem may be selectively found in a subgroup of deaf adolescents who perceive unfavorable social circumstances as an inescapable threat to their global self-worth (van Gent et al., 2012). As both deaf and hearing children tend to interact more intensely with age peers of similar hearing status, intervention programs have been developed to increase social interaction between deaf and hearing peers. Research on social skills interventions aimed at promoting social interaction and social play suggests a much more positive effect on interaction between deaf children than on interaction between deaf children and their hearing peers (Antia & Kreimeyer, 2003). By providing more opportunities to develop intense social connections between deaf and hearing peers, long-term and more intensive interventions (e.g., coenrollment programs) seem to have more and longer-lasting success than less intensive interventions (ibid.). Coenrollment or coteaching programs at schools where deaf and hearing peers learn together are jointly taught by a team consisting of a general education teacher, a teacher of deaf students, and an interpreter.

Children's sociocultural and linguistic background may affect their ability to understand their own and others' minds. Studies suggest that native signers (i.e., deaf children in households with signing deaf parents or at least one other native signer) perform comparably to hearing peers on a variety of tasks measuring theory of mind (TOM), which is the ability to attribute mental states to others as well as to oneself (Courtin & Melot, 1998; Peterson & Siegal, 1998, 2000; Meristo et al., 2007; Schick, De Villiers, De Villiers, & Hoffmeister, 2007). Early or native signers outperform those acquiring sign language later (e.g., deaf children of hearing parents) on both verbal and less verbal theory of mind (TOM) tasks (Courtin & Melot, 1998; Peterson et al., 2005; Meristo et al., 2007; Schick et al., 2007). This difference persists even after the effects of language ability, nonverbal mental age, and executive functioning have been taken into account (Woolfe, Want, & Siegal, 2002). However, longitudinal research on the sequential progression of TOM in deaf children suggests that those who missed early conversational inputs may continue to improve their understanding of TOM at advanced ages (Pyers & Senghas, 2009; Wellman, Fang, & Peterson, 2011). Thus, the pace of TOM development in deaf children is not associated with deafness in itself but rather with factors that influence the extent of linguistic and social attunement between caregivers and the deaf child such as the presence or absence of early access to a fluently shared common language (Peterson & Slaughter, 2006; Morgan & Kegl, 2006), early exposure to dyadic conversation about mental states (Meins et al., 2002; Moeller & Schick, 2006), a bilingual context (Goetz, 2003), or a normal course of experience with social interaction and conversation (Wellman et al., 2011) in general. Rieffe and Meerum-Terwogt (Meerum-Terwogt & Rieffe, 2004; Rieffe & Meerum-Terwogt, 2000) investigated deaf children's spontaneous negotiation strategies in false-belief situations. As compared to their hearing age peers, deaf children of hearing parents were found to use an abundance of references to their own desires and needs, combined with a lack of perspective taking. The authors suggest that an understanding of other people's emotions in deaf children may be hampered as a consequence of limited interaction with their hearing parents.

DEAF-BLIND CHILDREN

Epidemiology

Deaf-blindness is a serious multisensory impairment. Someone may be called deaf-blind when he or she has a combined loss of hearing and vision. The two together increase the effects of each (Sense, 2014). An estimated 0.01/1,000 children are deaf-blind (Best, 1983), but this is likely to be an underestimate (Hindley & van Gent, 2002). In the past, congenital rubella has accounted for one-third to one-half of cases (Trybus, 1985), but this has decreased as a result of widespread rubella immunization in many countries. Both genetic conditions such as Usher syndrome and CHARGE syndrome (an acronym for the combination of coloboma, heart defects, choanal atresia, retardation of growth after birth, genital hypoplasia, and ear malformations) and deafness in the majority of cases (Verloes, 2005; Pauli, Steckel, Zoll, & Wehner, 2006), as well as nongenetic conditions such as brain abnormalities associated with very low birth weight, are now likely to account for the majority. In general, additional impairments are very common: Intellectual impairment occurs in one-third to one-half, brain abnormalities in one-quarter of all cases (Trybus, 1985), and psychosis in about 13% of people with congenital deaf-blindness (Dammeyer, 2011). The impact of deaf-blindness greatly depends on the timing and progression of the respective losses of vision and hearing, as well as the order of appearance. The psychological balance between carrying capacity and the burden the child carries is totally different for a child who is born deaf-blind and has a concomitant cognitive impairment as a result of CNS damage due to intra-uterine rubella infection than it is for a child born deaf, having balance problems, and becoming progressively visually restricted due to Usher syndrome, the most common cause of deaf-blindness (1/10,000). Often the latter children develop night blindness at about the age of 10 years, followed by progressive peripheral vision loss in puberty, resulting in increased anxiety and sense of isolation as they face the progressive loss of vision during this phase of development.

Impact of Multisensory Impairment

Deaf-blindness is one of the most devastating (Adler, 1987) and least understood of handicapping conditions (McInnes & Treffry, 1982). Deaf-blind children and young people face challenges that are often greater than the sum of the hearing and visual impairments because sensory information needs to be integrated. Their main difficulties lie in accessing experience as such, and that experience often has to be mediated through others. However, the impact of deaf-blindness on children and their families is influenced by the severity of the sensory impairments and the nature and severity of associated impairments (Jenkins & Chess, 1996). Responses to sensory losses may include feelings of anxiety, isolation, denial, resentment, or distortion of body image (Adler, 1987; Hindley & van Gent, 2002). Children with a multisensory impairment require enormous adaptation on the part of their parents (McInnes & Treffry, 1982). In the case of Usher syndrome, many parents appear devastated and unable to imagine the future life of their child when they are informed that their already deaf child may well go progressively blind (Miner, 1995).

Cultural Aspects

In areas where the incidence of Usher syndrome is high (e.g., in the Cajun community of Louisiana), deaf-blind communities have formed. A similar community has formed in Seattle, Washington, primarily through migration. Miner (1999) provided essential guidance on therapeutic techniques when working with deaf-blind people (see also the website www.deafblind.com).

REFERENCES

Adler, M. A. (1987). Psychosocial interventions with deaf-blind youths and adults. In B. W. Heller, L. M. Flohr, & L. S. Zegans (Eds.), *Psychosocial interventions with sensorially disabled persons* (pp. 187–207). London: Grune & Stratton.

Antia, S. D., Jones, P. B., Reed, S., & Kreimeyer, K. H. (2009). Academic status and progress of deaf and hard-of-hearing students in general education classrooms. *Journal of Deaf Studies and Deaf Education, 14,* 293–311.

Antia, S. D., & Kreimeyer, K. (2003). Peer interactions of deaf and hard of hearing children. In M. Marschark & P. E. Spencer (Eds.), *Oxford handbook of deaf studies, language, and education* (pp. 164–176). New York: Oxford University Press.

Antia, S. D., Kreimeyer, K. H., & Eldridge, N. (1993). Promoting social interaction between young children with hearing impairments and their peers. *Exceptional Children, 60,* 262–275.

Armstrong, D. F., & Wilcox, S. (2003). Origins of sign languages. In M. Marschark & P. E. Spencer (Eds.), *Oxford handbook of deaf studies, language, and education* (pp. 305–318). New York: Oxford University Press.

Baker, A. (2007). *Taal- en spraakontwikkeling: Nieuwe inzichten.* Lezing Boerhaave cursus kinder- en jeugdpsychiatrie [Language and speech development: New Insights. Lecture Boerhaave course on child and adolescent psychiatry], September 20, Leiden.

Baker, S. A., Michnick Golinkoff, R., & Petitto, L. A. (2006). New insights into old puzzles from infants' categorical discrimination of soundless phonetic units. *Language Learning and Development, 2,* 147–162.

Bat-Chava, Y., Martin, D., & Kosciw, J. G. (2004). Longitudinal improvements in communication and socialization of deaf children with cochlear implants and hearing aids: Evidence from parental reports. *Journal of Child Psychology and Psychiatry, 46,* 1287–1296.

Beadle, E. A. R., McKinley, D. J., Nikolopoulos, T. P., Brough, J., O'Donoghue, G. M., & Archibold, S. M. (2005). Long-term functional outcomes and academic-occupational status in implanted children after 10 to 14 years of cochlear implant use. *Otology & Neurotology, 26,* 1152–1160.

Bellugi, U., O'Grady, L., Lillo-Martin, D., Hynes, M. O., Van Hoek, K., & Corina, D. (1990). Enhancement of spatial cognition in deaf children. In V. Volterra & C. J. Erting (Eds.), *From gesture to language in hearing and deaf children* (pp. 278–298). New York: Springer.

Best, C. (1983). The "new" deaf-blind? Results of a national survey of deaf-blind children in ESN(S) and hospital schools. *British Journal of Visual Impairment, 1,* 11–13.

Bettger, J. G., Emmorey, K., McCullough, S. H., & Bellugi, U. (1997). Enhanced facial discrimination: Effects of experience with American Sign Language. *Journal of Deaf Studies and Deaf Education, 2,* 223–233.

Bialystok, E. (2007). Cognitive effects of bilingualism: How linguistic experience leads to cognitive change. *International Journal of Bilingual Education and Bilingualism, 10,* 210–223.

Bialystok, E. (2011). Reshaping the mind: The benefits of bilingualism. *Canadian Journal of Experimental Psychology, 15,* 229–235.

Bialystok, E., & Craik, F. I. M. (2010). Cognitive and linguistic processing in the bilingual mind. *Current Directions in Psychological Science, 19,* 19–23.

Blamey, P. J., Sarant, J. Z., Paatsch, L. E., Barry, J. G., Bow, C. P., Wales, R. J., Wright, M., Psarros, C., Rattigan, K., & Toolher, R. (2001). Perceptions among speech perception, production, language, hearing loss, and age in children with impaired hearing. *Journal of Speech, Language, and Hearing Research, 44,* 264–285.

Blennerhassett, L. (2000). Psychological assessments. In P. Hindley & N. Kitson (Eds.), *Mental health and deafness* (pp. 185–205). London: Whurr.

Braden, J. P. (1994). *Deafness, deprivation and IQ.* New York: Plenum.

Calderon, R., & Greenberg, M. T. (1993). Considerations in the adaptation of families with school-aged deaf children. In M. Marschark & D. Clark (Eds.), *Psychological perspectives on deafness* (pp. 27–48). Hillsdale, NJ: Erlbaum.

Calderon, R., & Greenberg, M. T. (1999). Stress and coping in hearing mothers of children with hearing loss: Factors affecting mother and child adjustment. *American Annals of the Deaf, 144,* 7–18.

Calderon, R., & Greenberg, M. T. (2003). Social and emotional development of deaf children: Family, school and program effects. In M. Marschark & P. E. Spencer (Eds.), *Oxford handbook of deaf studies, language, and education* (pp. 177–189). New York: Oxford University Press.

Campbell, R. (1998). Read the lips: Speculation on the nature and role of lipreading in cognitive development of deaf children. In M. Marschark, P. Siple, D. Lillo-Martin, R. Campbell, & V. Everhart (Eds.), *Relations of language and thought: The view from sign language and deaf children* (pp. 110–146). Oxford: Oxford University Press.

Campbell, R., MacSweeney, M., & Waters, D. (2008). Sign language and the brain: A review. *Journal of Deaf Studies and Deaf Education, 13,* 3–20.

Capelli, M., Daniels, T., Durieux-Smith, McGrath, P. J., & Neuss, D. (1995). Social development of children with hearing impairments who are integrated into general education classrooms. *Volta Review, 97,* 197–208.

Caselli, M. C., & Volterra, V. (1989). From communication to language in hearing and deaf children. In V. Volterra & C. J. Erting (Eds.), *From Gesture to language in hearing and deaf children* (pp. 263–277). Berlin: Springer.

Christiansen, J., & Leigh, I. (2004). *Cochlear implants in children: Ethics and choices.* Washington, DC: Gallaudet University Press.

Connor, C., Hieber, S., Arts, A., & Zwolan, T. (2000). Speech, vocabulary, and the education of children using cochlear implants: Oral or total communication? *Journal of Speech, Language, and Hearing Research, 43,* 1185–1204.

Corina, D. P. (1999). Neural disorders of language and movement: Evidence from American Sign Language. In L. Messing & R. Campbell (Eds.), *Gesture, speech, and sign* (pp. 27–44). Oxford: Oxford University Press.

Corina, D. P., & Singleton, J. (2009). Developmental social neuroscience: Insights from deafness. *Child Development, 80,* 952–967.

Courtin, C., & Melot, A. M. (1998). Development of theories of mind in deaf children. In M. Marschark & M. D. Clarke (Eds.), *Psychological perspectives of deafness, Vol. 2* (pp. 79–102). Mahwah, NJ: Erlbaum.

Dammeyer, J. (2011). Mental and behavioral disorders among people with congenital blindness. *Research in Developmental Disabilities, 32,* 572–575.

Danek, M. M. (1988). Deafness and family impact. In P. Power, A. Sell Orto, & M. Gibsons (Eds.), *Family interventions throughout chronic illness and disability* (pp. 120–135). New York: Springer.

Davis, A., & Parving, A. (1994). Towards appropriate epidemiology data on childhood hearing disability: A comparative European study of birth cohorts 1982–88. *Journal of Audiologic Medicine, 3*, 35–47.

De Graaf, R., Knippers, E. W. A., & Bijl, R. (1997). Prevalentie en relevante achtergrond-kenmerken van doofheid en ernstige slechthorendheid in Nederland [Prevalence and relevant background characteristics of deafness and severe hardness of hearing in the Netherlands]. *Nederlands Tijdschrift voor Geneeskunde, 142*, 1819–1823.

Emmorey, K., & Kosslyn, S. (1996). Enhanced image generation abilities in deaf signers: A right hemisphere effect. *Brain and Cognition, 32*, 28–44.

Emmorey, K., Kosslyn, S., & Bellugi, U. (1993). Visual imagery and visual-spatial language: Enhanced imagery abilities in deaf and hearing ASL signers. *Cognition, 46*, 139–181.

Erting, C. J. (1982). *Deafness, communication and social identity: An anthropological analysis of interaction among parents, teachers and deaf children in preschool.* Unpublished dissertation, American University, Washington, DC.

Erting, C. J., Prezioso, C., & O'Grady Hynes, M. (1989). The interactional context of deaf mother-infant interactions. In V. Volterra & C. J. Erting (Eds.), *From gesture to language in hearing and deaf children* (pp. 97–106). Berlin: Springer.

Farrugia, D., & Austin, G. F. (1980). A study of social-emotional adjustment patterns of hearing-impaired students in different educational settings. *American Annals of the Deaf, 125*, 535–541.

Feinstein, C. B. (1983). Early adolescent deaf boys: A biopsychosocial approach. *Adolescent Psychiatry, 11*, 147–162.

Fortnum, H. M., & Davis, A. (1997). Epidemiology of permanent childhood hearing impairment in Trent region. *British Journal of Audiology, 31*, 409–496.

Fortnum, H. M., Marshall, D. H., & Summerfield, A. Q. (2002). Epidemiology of the United Kingdom population of hearing-impaired children including characteristics of those with and without cochlear implants: Audiology, etiology, co-morbidity, and affluence. *International Journal of Audiology, 41*, 170–179.

Fortnum, H. M., Summerfield, A. Q., Marshall, D. H., Davis, A. C., & Bamford, J. M. (2001). Prevalence of permanent childhood hearing impairment in the United Kingdom and implications for neonatal hearing screening: questionnaire based ascertainment study. *British Medical Journal, 323*, 1–5.

Freeman, R. D., Malkin, S. F., & Hastings, J. O. (1975). Psychological problems of deaf children and their families: A comparative study. *American Annals of the Deaf, 120*, 275–304.

Goldin-Meadow, S. (2010). Widening the lens on language learning: Language creation in deaf children and adults in Nicaragua. Commentary on Senghas. *Human Development, 53*, 303–311.

Goetz, P. J. (2003). The effects of bilingualism on theory of mind development. *Bilingualism: Language and Cognition, 6*, 1–15.

Gorlin, R. J., Toriello, H. V., & Cohen, M. M. (Eds.). (1995). *Hereditary hearing loss and its syndromes.* New York: Oxford University Press.

Greenberg, M. T., & Kusché, M. T. (1993). *Promoting social and emotional development in deaf children: The PATHS Project.* Seattle: University of Washington Press.

Groce, N. E., & Whiting, M. (1988). *Everyone here spoke sign language: Hereditary deafness on Martha's Vineyard.* Cambridge, MA: Harvard University Press.

Haggard, M., & Hughes, E. (1991). *Screening of children's hearing: A review of the literature and the implications of OM.*, London: HMSO.

Harris, M. (2000). Social interaction and early language development in deaf children. *Deafness & Education International, 2*, 1–11.

Harris, M. (2001). It's all a matter of timing: Sign visibility and sign reference in deaf and hearing mothers of 18-month-old children. *Journal of Deaf Studies and Deaf Education, 6*, 177–185.

Harris, R. I. (1978). The relationship of impulse control to parent hearing status, manual communication and academic achievement in deaf children. *American Annals of the Deaf, 123*, 52–67.

Hauser, P. C., Lukomski, J., & Hillman, T. (2008). Development of deaf and hard-of-hearing students' executive function. In M. Marschark & P. C. Hauser (Eds.), *Deaf cognition: Foundations and outcomes* (pp. 286–308). Oxford: Oxford University Press.

Hauser, P. C., & Marschark, M. (2008). What we know and what we don't know about cognition and deaf learners. In M. Marschark & P. C. Hauser (Eds.), *Deaf cognition: Foundations and outcomes* (pp. 439–457). Oxford: Oxford University Press.

Hindley, P. A. (1997). Psychiatric aspects of hearing impairments. *Journal of Child Psychology and Psychiatry, 38*, 101–117.

Hindley, P. A. (1999). The cultural-linguistic model of deafness: response by a psychodynamic family psychiatrist specializing in work with families which include a deaf child. *Journal of Social Work Practice, 13*, 174–176.

Hindley, P. A., & van Gent, T. (2002). Psychiatric aspects of specific hearing impairments. In M. Rutter & E. Taylor (Eds.), *Child and adolescent psychiatry* (4th ed.) (pp. 842–857). Oxford: Blackwell Science.

Hintermair, M. (2007). Prevalence of socioemotional problems in deaf and hard of hearing children in Germany. *American Annals of the Deaf, 152*, 320–330.

Hoffmeister, R., de Villiers, P., Engen, E., & Topol, D. (1997). English reading achievement and ASL skills in deaf students. In E. Hughes, M. Hughes, & A. Greenhill (Eds.), *Proceedings of the 21st Annual Boston University Conference on Language Development* (pp. 307–318). Somerville, MA: Cascadilla Press.

Jenkins, I. R., & Chess, S. (1996). Psychiatric evaluation of perceptually impaired children: Hearing and visual impairments. In M. Lewis (Ed.), *Child and adolescent psychiatry: A comprehensive textbook* (2nd ed.) (pp. 526–534). Baltimore: Williams and Wilkins.

Kegl, J., Senghas, A., & Coppola, M. (1999). Creation through contact: Sign language emergence and sign language change in Nicaragua. In M. DeGraff (Ed.), *Language creation and language change: Creolization, diachrony, and development* (pp. 179–237). Cambridge, MA: MIT Press.

Kluwin, T. N. (1999). Co-teaching deaf and hearing students: Research on social integration. *American Annals of the Deaf, 144*, 339–344.

Kluwin, T. N., Stinson, M. S., & Colarossi, G. M. (2002) Social processes and outcomes of in-school contact between deaf and hearing peers. *Journal of Deaf Studies and Deaf Education, 7*, 200–213.

Knoors, H., & Marschark, M. (2012, Summer). Language planning for the 21st century: Revisiting bilingual language policy for deaf children. *Journal of Deaf Studies and Deaf Education, 17*(3), 291–305. doi: 10.1093/deafed/ens018

Koester, L. S. (1994). Early interactions and the socioemotional development of deaf infants. *Early Development and Parenting, 3*, 51–60.

Korver, A. M. H., Admiraal, R. J. C., Kant, S. G., Dekker, F. W., Wever, C. C., Kunst, H. P. M., Frijns, J. H. M., & Oudesluys-Murphy, A. M. (2011). Causes of permanent childhood hearing impairment. *Laryngoscope, 121*, 409–416.

Krentz, U. C., & Corina, D. P. (2008). Preference for language in early infancy: The human language bias is not speech specific. *Developmental Science, 11*, 1–9.

Kusché, C. A., Greenberg, M. T., & Garfield, T. S. (1983). Nonverbal intelligence and verbal achievement in deaf adolescents: An examination of heredity and environment. *American Annals of the Deaf, 128*, 458–466.

Lederberg, A., & Mobley, C. (1990). The effect of hearing impairment on the quality of attachment and mother toddler interaction. *Child Development, 61,* 1596–1604.

Lederberg, A., Ryan, H. B., & Robbins, B. L. (1986). Peer interaction in young deaf children: The effect of partner hearing status and familiarity. *Developmental Psychology, 22,* 691–700.

Loots, G., & Devisé, I. (2003). The use of visual-tactile communication strategies by deaf and hearing fathers and mothers of deaf infants. *Journal of Deaf Studies and Deaf Education, 8,* 31–42.

Loots, G., Devisé, I., & Jacquet, W. (2005). The impact of visual communication on the intersubjective development of early parent-child interaction with 18- to 24-month-old deaf toddlers. *Journal of Deaf Studies and Deaf Education, 10,* 357–375.

MacSweeney, M., Woll, B., Campbell, R., Calvert, G. A., McGuire, P. K., David, A. S., Simmons, A., & Brammer, M. J. (2002). Neural correlates of British sign language comprehension: Spatial processing demands of topographic language. *Journal of Cognitive Neuroscience, 14,* 1064–1075.

Maller, S. J. (2003). Intellectual assessment of deaf people: A critical review of core concepts and issues. In M. Marschark & P. E. Spencer (Eds.), *Oxford handbook of deaf studies, language, and education* (pp. 451–463). Oxford: Oxford University Press.

Marschark, M. (1993). *Psychological development of deaf children.* Oxford: Oxford University Press.

Marschark, M. (2003). Cognitive functioning in deaf adults and children. In M. Marschark & P. E. Spencer (Eds.), *Oxford handbook of deaf studies, language, and education* (pp. 464–477). Oxford: Oxford University Press.

Marschark, M. (2007). *Raising and educating a deaf child* (2nd ed.). Oxford: Oxford University Press.

Marschark, M., & Wauters, L. (2008). Language comprehension and learning by deaf students. In M. Marschark & P. C. Hauser (Eds.). *Deaf cognition: Foundations and outcomes* (pp. 309–350). Oxford: Oxford University Press.

Masataka, N. (1996). Perception of motherese in a signed language by 6-month-old deaf infants. *Developmental Psychology, 32,* 874–879.

Masataka, N. (2003). *The onset of language.* Cambridge: Cambridge University Press.

Maxwell-McCaw, D., & Zea, M. C. (2011). The Deaf acculturation scale (DAS): Development and validation of a 58-item measure. *Journal of Deaf Studies and Deaf Education, 16,* 325–342.

Mayberry, R. I. (2002). Cognitive development in deaf children: The interface of language and perception in neuropsychology. In S. J. Segalowitz & I. Rapin (Eds.), *Handbook of neuropsychology* (2nd ed.), *Vol. 8,* part 2 (pp. 71–107). Amsterdam: Elsevier Science.

Mayberry, R. I., Lock, E., & Kazmi, H. (2002). Linguistic ability and early language exposure. *Nature, 417,* 38.

McCullough, S., & Emmorey, K. (1997). Face processing by deaf ASL signers: Evidence for expertise in distinguishing local features. *Journal of Deaf Studies and Deaf Education, 2,* 212–222.

McInnes, J. M., & Treffry, J. A. (1982). *Deaf-blind infants and children: A developmental guide.* Milton Keynes, UK: Open University Press.

Meadow-Orlans, K. (1995). Parenting with a sensory or physical disability. In M. Borstein (Ed.), *Handbook of parenting: Vol. 4, Applied and practical considerations* (pp. 57–84). Hillsdale, NJ: Erlbaum.

Meadow-Orlans, K. P., & Erting, C. (2000). Deaf people in society. In P. Hindley & N. Kitson (Eds.), *Mental health and deafness* (pp. 3–24). London: Whurr.

Meerum-Terwogt, M., & Rieffe, C. (2004). Deaf children's use of beliefs and desires in nego-tiation. *Journal of Deaf Studies and Deaf Education, 9,* 27–38.

Meins, E., Fernyhough, C., Wainwright, R., Gupta, M. D., Fradley, R., & Tuckey, M. (2002). Maternal mind-mindedness and attachment security as predictors of theory of mind understanding. *Child Development, 73,* 1715–1726.

Meristo, M., Falkman, K. W., Hjelmquist, E., Tedoldi, M., Surian, L., & Siegal, M. (2007). Language access and theory of mind reasoning: Evidence from deaf children in bilingual and oralist environments. *Developmental Psychology, 43,* 1156–1169.

Meyer, T. A., Svirsky, M. A., Kirk, K. I., & Miyamoto, R. T. (1998). Improvements in speech perception by children with profound hearing loss: Effects of device, communica-tion, mode and chronological age. *Journal of Speech, Language and Hearing Research, 41,* 846–848.

Miner, I. D. (1995). Psychosocial implications of Usher syndrome, type I, throughout the life cycle. *Journal of Visual Impairment and Blindness, 89,* 287–296.

Miner, I. D. (1999). Psychotherapy for people with Usher syndrome. In I. W. Leigh (Ed.), *Psychotherapy with deaf clients from diverse client groups* (pp. 302–327). Washington, DC: Gallaudet University Press.

Miyahara. M., & Piek, J. (2006). Self-esteem of children and adolescents with physical dis-abilities: Quantitative evidence from meta-analysis. *Journal of Development and Physical Disabilities, 18,* 219–234.

Moeller, M. P. (2000). Early intervention and language development in children who are deaf and hard of hearing. *Pediatrics, 106,* 1–9.

Moeller, M. P., & Schick, B. (2006). Relations between maternal input and theory of mind understanding in deaf children. *Child Development, 77,* 751–766.

Morford, J. P. (1998). Gesture when there is no speech model. *New Directions for Child Devel-opment, 79,* 101–116.

Morgan, G., & Kegl, J. (2006). Nicaraguan sign language and theory of mind: The issue of critical periods and abilities. *Journal of Child Psychology and Psychiatry, 47,* 811–819.

Neville, H. J., & Lawson, D. (1987). Attention to central and peripheral visual space in a movement detection task: An event-related potential and behavioral study. II: Con-genitally deaf adults. *Brain Research, 405,* 268–283.

Newport, E. L., Bavelier, D., & Neville, H. J. (2001). Critical thinking about critical peri-ods: Perspectives on a critical period for language acquisition. In E. Dupoux (Ed.), *Language, brain and cognitive development: Essays in honour of Jacques Mehler* (pp. 481–502). Cambridge, MA: MIT Press.

Padden, C., & Ramsey, C. (1998). Reading ability in signing deaf children. In *Topics in Lan-guage Disorders: ASL Proficiency and English Literacy Acquisition: New Perspectives, 18,* 30–46.

Pauli, S., Steckel, M., Zoll, B., & Wehner, L.-E. (2006). CHARGE: Von einer Assoziation zum Syndrom [CHARGE: From association to syndrome]. *Monatsschrift Kinderheilkunde, 1,* 23–28.

Peterson, C. C., & Siegal, M. (1998). Changing focus on the representational mind: Deaf, autistic and normal children's concepts of false photos, false drawings & false beliefs. *British Journal of Developmental Psychology, 16,* 301–320.

Peterson, C. C., & Siegal, M. (2000). Insights into theory of mind from deafness and autism. *Mind & Language, 15,* 123–145.

Peterson, C. C., & Slaughter, V. P. (2006). Telling the story of theory of mind: Deaf and hear-ing children's narratives and mental state understanding. *British Journal of Developmen-tal Psychology, 24,* 151–179.

Peterson, C. C., Wellman, H. M., & Liu, D. (2005). Steps in theory-of-mind development for children with deafness or autism. *Child Development, 76,* 502–517.

Petitto, L. A., Holowka, S., Sergio, L. E., Levy, B., & Ostry, D. J. (2004). Baby hands that move to the rhythm of language: Hearing babies acquiring sign languages babble silently on the hands. *Cognition, 93,* 43–73.

Petitto, L. A., & Marentette, P. F. (1991). Babbling in the manual mode: Evidence for the ontogeny of language. *Science, 251,* 1493–1496.

Pipp-Siegel, S., Sedey, A. L., & Yoshinaga-Itano, C. (2002). Predictors of parental stress on mothers of young children with hearing loss. *Journal of Deaf Studies and Deaf Education, 7,* 1–17.

Power, D. J., Wood, D. J., & Wood, H. A. (1990). Conversational strategies of teachers using three methods of communication with deaf children. *American Annals of the Deaf, 135,* 9–13.

Prendergast, S. G., & McCollum, J. A. (1996). Let's talk: The effect of maternal hearing status on interactions with toddlers who are deaf. *American Annals of the Deaf, 141,* 11–18.

Pressman, L., Pipp-Siegel, S., Yoshinaga-Itano, C., Kubicek, L., & Emde, R. N. (2000). A comparison of the link between emotional availability and language gain in young children with and without hearing loss. *Volta Review, 100,* 251–277.

Prinz, P., & Strong, M. (1998). ASL proficiency and English literacy within a bilingual deaf education model of instruction. *Topical Language Disorders, 18,* 47–60.

Proksch, J., & Bavelier, D. (2002). Changes in the spatial distribution of visual attention after early deafness. *Journal of Cognitive Neuroscience, 14,* 687–701.

Punch, R., & Hyde, M. (2011). Social participation of children and adolescents with cochlear implants: A qualitative analysis of parent, teacher, and child interviews. *Journal of Deaf Studies and Deaf Education, 16,* 474–493.

Pyers, J., & Sengas, A. (2009). Language promotes false-belief understanding: Evidence from a new sign language. *Psychological Science, 20,* 805–812.

Quigley, S., & Paul, P. (1984). *Language and deafness.* San Diego: College-Hill Press.

Rieffe, C., & Meerum Terwogt, M. (2000). Deaf children's understanding of emotions: Desires take precedence. *Journal of Child Psychology and Psychiatry, 41,* 601–608.

Rönnberg, J., Söderfeldt, B., & Risberg, J. (2000). The cognitive neuroscience of signed language. *Acta Psychologica, 105,* 237–254.

Sass-Lehrer, M., & Bodner-Johnson, B. (2003). Early intervention: Current approaches to family-centered programming. In M. Marschark & P. E. Spencer (Eds.), *Oxford handbook of deaf studies, language, and education* (pp. 65–81). Oxford: Oxford University Press.

Schick, B. (2003). The development of American sign language and manually coded English systems. In M. Marschark & P. E. Spencer (Eds.), *Oxford handbook of deaf studies, language, and education* (pp. 219–231). Oxford: Oxford University Press.

Schick, B., De Villiers, P., De Villiers, J., & Hoffmeister, R. (2007). Language and theory of mind: A study of deaf children. *Child Development, 78,* 376–396.

Senghas, A. (2010). The emergence of two functions for spatial devices in Nicaraguan sign language. *Human Development, 53,* 287–302.

Sense (2014). About deafblindness. http://www.sense.org.uk/content/about-deafblindess

Singleton, J. L., & Tittle, M. D. (2000). Deaf parents and their hearing children. *Journal of Deaf Studies and Deaf Education, 5,* 221–236.

Sinkkonen, J. (1994). *Hearing impairment, communication and personality development.* Unpublished doctoral dissertation, University of Helsinki.

Sisco, F. H., & Anderson, R. J. (1980). Deaf children's performance on the WISC-R relative to hearing status of parents and child-rearing experiences. *American Annals of the Deaf, 125,* 923–930.

Smith, S., & Koester, L. S. (1995). Defining and observing social signals in deaf and hearing infants. *American Annals of the Deaf, 140,* 422–427.

Snitzer Reilly, J., McIntire, M. L., & Bellugi, U. (1989). Faces: The relationship between language and affect. In V. Volterra & C. J. Erting (Eds.), *From gesture to language in hearing and deaf children* (pp. 128–141). Berlin: Springer-Verlag.

Spencer, L. J., Gantz, B. J., & Knutson. (2004). Outcomes and achievement of students who grew up with access to cochlear implants. *Laryngoscope, 114,* 1576–1581.

Spencer, P. E., Bodner-Johnson, B. A., & Gutfreund, M. (1992). Interacting with infants with a hearing loss: What can we learn from mothers who are deaf? *Journal of Early Intervention, 16,* 64–78.

Spencer, P. E., & Marschark, M. (2003). Cochlear implants: Issues and implications. In M. Marschark & P. E. Spencer (Eds.), *Oxford handbook of deaf studies, language, and education* (pp. 434–448). Oxford: Oxford University Press.

Spencer, P. E., & Meadow-Orlans, K. P. (1996). Play, language and maternal responsiveness: A longitudinal study of deaf and hearing infants. *Child Development, 67,* 3176–3191.

Steinberg, A. (2000). Autobiographical narrative on growing up deaf. In P. E. Spencer & M. Marschark (Eds.), *The deaf child in the family and at school: Essays in honor of Kathryn P. Meadow-Orlans* (pp. 93–108). Mahwah, NJ: Erlbaum.

Stephens, D. (2001). Audiometric investigation in first-degree relatives. In A. Martini, M. Mazzolli, D. Stephens, & A. Read (eds.), *Definitions, protocols and guidelines in genetic hearing impairment* (pp. 32–33). London: Whurr.

Stinson, M. S., & Kluwin, T. N. (2003). Educational consequences of alternative school placements. In M. Marschark & P. E. Spencer (Eds.), *Oxford handbook of deaf studies, language, and education* (pp. 52–64). Oxford: Oxford University Press.

Stokoe, W. (1998). A very long perspective. In M. Marschark & M. D. Clarke (Eds.), *Psychological perspectives on deafness* (2nd ed.) (pp. 1–18). Mahwah, NJ: Erlbaum.

Supalla, S. (1991). Manually coded English: The modality question in signed language development. In P. Siple & S. D. Fischer (Eds.), *Theoretical issues in sign language research: Vol. 2, Psychology* (pp. 86–109). Chicago: University of Chicago Press.

Sutton-Spence, R., & Woll, B. (1999). *The linguistics of British Sign Language: An introduction.* Cambridge: Cambridge University Press.

Talbot, K. F., & Haude, R. H. (1993). The relationship between sign language skill an spatial visualizations ability: Mental rotation of three dimensional objects. *Perceptual and Motor Skills, 77,* 1387–1391.

Traci, M., & Koester, L. S. (2003). Parent-infant interactions: A transactional approach to understanding the development of deaf infants. In M. Marschark & P. E. Spencer (Eds.), *Oxford handbook of deaf studies, language, and education* (pp. 190–202). New York: Oxford University Press.

Traxler, C. B. (2000). The Stanford Achievement Test, 9th edition: National norming and performance standards for deaf and hard-of-hearing students. *Journal of Deaf Studies and Deaf Education, 5,* 337–348.

Trybus, R. J. (1985). Demographics and population character research in deaf-blindness. In J. E. Stahlecker, L. E. Glass, & S. Machalow (Eds.), *State of the art: Research priorities in deaf-blindness.* San Francisco: University of California–San Francisco, Center on Deafness.

van Gent, T. (2012). Mental health problems in deaf children and adolescents. In T. van Gent, *Mental health problems in deaf and severely hard of hearing children and adolescents. Findings on prevalence, pathogenesis and clinical complexities, and implications for prevention, diagnosis and intervention* (pp. 23–80). PhD thesis, Leiden University, the Netherlands.

van Gent, T., Goedhart, A., Knoors, H., Westenberg, P. M., & Treffers, Ph. D. A. (2012, February 20). Self-concept and ego development in deaf adolescents: Associations with social context and deafness-related variables, and a comparison with hearing adolescents. *Journal of Deaf Studies and Deaf Education, 17*(3), 333–351, doi: 10.1093/deafed/ens002

van Gurp, S. (2001). Self-concept of secondary school students in different educational settings. *Journal of Deaf Studies and Deaf Education, 6,* 55–69.

Verloes, A. (2005). Updated diagnostic criteria for CHARGE syndrome: A proposal. *American Journal of Medical Genetics, 133A,* 306–308.

Vernon, M. (1968/2005). Fifty years of research on the intelligence of deaf and hard-of-hearing children: A review of literature and discussion of implications. *Journal of Rehabilitation of the Deaf, 1,* 1–12. (Reprinted in the *Journal of Deaf Studies and Deaf Education, 10,* 225–231).

Walch, C., Anderhuber, W., Köle, W., & Berghold, A. (2000). Bilateral sensorineural hearing disorders in children: Etiology of deafness and evaluation of hearing tests. *International Journal of Pediatric Otorhinolaryngology, 53,* 31–38.

Watkins, S., Pitman, P., & Walden, B. (1998). The deaf mentor experimental project for young children who are deaf and their families. *American Annals of the Deaf, 143,* 29–34.

Wellman, H. M., Fang, F., & Peterson, C. C. (2011). Sequential progressions in a theory-of-mind scale: Longitudinal perspectives. *Child Development, 82,* 780–792.

Wie, O. B., Falkenberg, E. S., Tvete, O., & Tomblin, B. (2007). Children with a cochlear implant: Characteristics and determinants of speech recognition, speech-recognition growth rate, and speech production. *International Journal of Audiology, 46,* 232–243.

Wood, D., Wood, H., Griffiths, A., & Howarth, I. (1986). *Teaching and talking with deaf children.* Chichester, West Sussex: John Wiley.

Woolfe, T., Want, S. C., & Siegal, M. (2002). Signpost to development: Theory of mind in deaf children. *Child Development, 73,* 768–778.

Yoshinaga-Itano, C. (2003). From screening to early identification and intervention: Discovering predictors to successful outcomes for children with significant hearing loss. *Journal of Deaf Studies and Deaf Education, 8,* 11–30.

Yoshinaga-Itano, C. (2006). Early identification, communication, and the development of speech and spoken language skills: Patterns and considerations. In P. E. Spencer & M. Marschark (Eds.), *Advances in spoken language development of deaf and hard of hearing children* (pp. 298–327). Oxford: Oxford University Press.

Yoshinaga-Itano, C., & Apuzzo M.-R. L. (1998). The development of deaf and hard of hearing children identified early through the high-risk registry. *American Annals of the Deaf, 143,* 416–424.

Young, A. M. (1999). Hearing parents adjustment to a deaf child: The impact of a cultural linguistic model of deafness. *Journal of Social Work Practice, 13,* 157–172.

Zwiebel, A. (1987). More on the effects of early manual communication on the cognitive development of deaf children. *American Annals of the Deaf, 134,* 16–22.

11

Mental Health Problems in Deaf Children and Adolescents: Part II—Aspects of Psychopathology

Tiejo van Gent

According to most studies, the incidence of psychopathology is greater in deaf children than in the general population, although the majority of these children do not have a mental disorder (Hindley, 1997). However, several mechanisms are likely to contribute to variations in the reported prevalence.

Methods of assessment and the choice of informants have varied from single-rating responses to questionnaires given to parents (Vostanis, Hayes, Du Feu, & Warren, 1997; van Eldik, Treffers, Veerman, & Verhulst, 2004; Hintermair, 2007) and teachers (Schlesinger & Meadow, 1972; Fundudis, Kolvin, & Garside, 1979; Aplin, 1985, 1987; Sinkkonen, 1994), self-reports (van Eldik, 2005; Cornes, Rohan, Napier, & Del Rey, 2006), ratings based on parental interviews (Fellinger, Holzinger, Sattel, Laucht, & Goldberg, 2009), two-stage designs combining information from parents and teachers with interview responses of deaf participants (Rutter, Graham, & Yule, 1970; Freeman, Malkin, & Hastings, 1975; Hindley, Hill, McGuigan, & Kitson, 1994) to one-stage, multiple-informant approaches incorporating relevant information from parents, teachers, deaf participants, clinicians, and medical files (van Gent, Goedhart, Hindley, & Treffers, 2007). Variations of

This chapter and the previous chapter by van Gent are updated and extended versions of T. van Gent, (2012), Mental health problems in deaf children and adolescents, in T. van Gent, *Mental health problems in deaf and severely hard of hearing children and adolescents. Findings on prevalence, pathogenesis and clinical complexities, and implications for prevention, diagnosis and intervention* (pp. 23–80), PhD thesis, Leiden University, Netherlands. The dissertation itself concerns a broadly renewed and adapted revision of P. A. Hindley & T. van Gent, (2002), Psychiatric aspects of specific hearing impairments, in M. Rutter & E. Taylor (Eds.), *Child and adolescent psychiatry* (4th ed.) (pp. 842–857). Oxford: Blackwell Science.

findings in studies using similar instruments and methods of calculating prevalence rates suggest that differences in the composition of the study samples contribute to differences in outcome. For instance, data from a small number of hearing
impaired participants ($N = 13$) in the whole population study by Rutter et al. (1970)
may lead to a relatively less reliable outcome. Furthermore, while most studies concentrated on both children and adolescents, some focused either on adolescents
(Hindley et al., 1994; van Eldik, 2005; Cornes et al., 2006; van Gent et al., 2007) or on
children (Fundudis et al., 1979), a factor that may have influenced the distribution
of disorders. For example, in one study more internalizing problems were found
among adolescents than among younger children (van Eldik et al., 2004), but in
other studies no significant age-related differences were found (Aplin, 1985, 1987).
Study samples also varied in two other characteristics: the degree of hearing loss
in the participants (table 1) and the type of school. Degree of hearing loss has been
associated with rate of psychopathology (Fundudis et al., 1979), but later studies do
not confirm this (Fellinger et al., 2009; Hintermair, 2007; van Eldik et al., 2004; van
Gent et al., 2007). The type of school may be more relevant to psychopathology than
degree of hearing loss (Hindley et al., 1994), as indicated in studies of students who
attended special schools for deaf children and adolescents (Aplin, 1985; Hintermair,
2007; Sinkkonen, 1994; van Eldik et al., 2004; Vostanis et al., 1997), ordinary school
only (Aplin, 1987) or more than one type of school (Fundudis et al., 1979; Hindley
et al., 1994; van Eldik, 2005; Cornes et al., 2006; van Gent et al., 2007).

Although some studies (Aplin, 1987; van Eldik, 2005) show that children in
mainstream schools display lower levels of mental health problems than do those
attending special schools, other factors (e.g., IQ, communication mode, physical
health) (van Gent et al., 2007) and referral bias (Hindley et al., 1994; van Gent et al.,
2007) may influence such conclusions. Findings are inconclusive as to whether disorders are more common among deaf children in mainstream or special schools.
Both deaf children in mainstream schools (Smith & Sharp, 1994) and deaf children in
special schools (Kouwenberg, Rieffe, Theunissen & de Rooij, 2012) were found to be
particularly at risk of being bullied. On the other hand, deaf children in residential
schools may be more vulnerable to abuse (Sullivan, Brookhouser, & Scanlan, 2000).

Finally, discrepancies in findings may be related to the extent to which instruments and assessment procedures have been adapted for use with deaf people.
Recent studies with such adaptations (Youth Self-Report [YSR]; see van Eldik, 2005;
Cornes, 2006) have found comparably increased prevalence rates (see table 1). The
range of psychiatric disorders in deaf children and adolescents is the same as in
their hearing peers (Hindley et al., 1994). Deaf children are exposed to a number of
additional risk factors, including communication problems, central nervous system disorders, physical health problems, and intellectual impairment (van Gent
et al., 2007; Hindley, 1997; Kammerer, 1988).

Findings from a Dutch study of a representative sample of deaf children and
adolescents who were referred to the national specialist mental health service over

TABLE 1. Studies of Prevalence of Mental Health Problems in Children and Adolescents with Hearing Impairment (HI) and Hearing Controls

1. Hearing impairment range (decibel loss in the unaided better ear): D = deaf without further specification; HH = hard of hearing without further specification; HI 1 = mild (20–40 dB); HI 2 = moderate (41–70 dB); HI 3 = severe (71–95 dB); HI 4 = profound (≥ 95 dB).

2. Assessment methods: I = psychiatric interview; O = psychiatric observation; R = Rutter scales (Rutter, Graham, & Yule, 1970); PCL = parent's checklist; TCL = teacher's checklist (Hindley et al. 1994); SDQ = Strengths and Difficulties Questionnaire (Goodman, 1997); combined = interviews in subjects screened positive; expert rating = multi-informant expert rating of caseness and diagnosis.

3. Data given in order of method of assessment or category of HI.

| Study | HI Sample: Number, Age Range, & Range of HI[1] | Methods of Assessment[2] | | | | | Prevalence of Mental Health Problems or Disorders | |
		Child	Parents	Teacher	Clinician	Measure	HI Sample (%)[3]	Hearing Control or Norm Group (%)
Rutter et al. (1970)	13; 5–14 years; HI 2–4	I	I+R	R		combined	15	7
Freeman et al. (1975)	115; 5–15 years; HI 3–4	O	I+R	R		combined	23	–
Fundudis et al. (1979)	54; 7–10 years; HI D/HH			R			Deaf: 54 / HH: 28	18
Aplin (1985)	61; 7–15 years; HI 1–4			R			36	–

(continued)

169

TABLE 1. Studies of Prevalence of Mental Health Problems in Children and Adolescents with Hearing Impairment (HI) and Hearing Controls *(continued)*

Study	HI Sample: Number, Age Range, & Range of HI[1]	Methods of Assessment[2]					Prevalence of Mental Health Problems or Disorders	
		Child	Parents	Teacher	Clinician	Measure	HI Sample (%)[3]	Hearing Control or Norm Group (%)
Aplin (1987)	42; 7–16 years; HI 1–4			R			17	–
Kammerer (1988)	183; 10–13 years; HI 1–4		I				54	–
Arnold et al. (1991)	23; 4–10 years; HI D/HH			R			0	–
Hindley et al. (1994)	81; 11–16 years; HI 2–4	I	I+PCL		TCL	combined	Deaf: 42 / HH unit: 61	–
Sinkkonen (1994)	294; 6–16 years; HI D/HH			R			Deaf: 19 / HH: 25	16
Mitchell et al. (1996)	39; 6–14 years; HI 3–4		CBCL	TRF			48 / 35	–
Vostanis et al. (1997)	84; 2–18 years; HI 3–4		CBCL/ PCL				43 / 77	–
van Eldik et al. (2004)	238; 4–18 years; HI 3–4		CBCL				41	16

(continued)

Study	HI Sample: Number, Age Range, & Range of HI[1]	Methods of Assessment[2]					Prevalence of Mental Health Problems or Disorders	
		Child	Parents	Teacher	Clinician	Measure	HI Sample (%)[3]	Hearing Control or Norm Group (%)
van Eldik (2005)	110; 11–18 years; HI 3–4	YSR					37	16
Cornes et al. (2006)	54; 11–18y; HI 3–4	YSR					43	19
van Gent et al. (2007)	68; 13–21 years; HI 3–4	I	CBCL	TRF	I	Expert rating	63 / 28 / 32 / 49 / 46	CBCL 16 / TRF 17
Hintermair (2007)	213; 4–13 years; HI D/HH		SDQ				36	15
Fellinger et al. (2009)	95; 6–16 years; HI 2–4		I				33	

a longer period of time (van Gent, Goedhart, & Treffers, 2012) illustrate the complexity of, and the need for, effective interventions, such as those aimed at early identification. As compared to hearing referrals from a large control group, deaf children and adolescents were on average referred at an older age and were subject to higher rates of environmental distress, as indicated by increased rates of parental divorce and one-parent families or lower parental educational level. In addition, higher rates of autism spectrum disorder, mental retardation, and disabling physical health conditions were found within the target group of the deaf referrals.

PSYCHIATRIC ASSESSMENT

During interviews of deaf children who rely on visual communication, the room needs to be uncluttered and well lit but without a bright light, such as a window behind the interviewer. Lipreading requires a clear view of the lips, and facial obstacles (e.g., bushy beards, moustaches, objects in the visual space between interviewer and interviewee) can cause problems (van Gent, 2000). No more than 25% of spoken language is seen through lip patterns alone (Conrad, 1979). Deaf people have to make educated guesses when lipreading (Beck & de Jong, 1990), and a strong foreign accent can make that even more difficult (Hindley & van Gent, 2002).

One of the primary goals for clinicians should be to minimize the impact of language barriers during the assessment and treatment process (Mathos & Broussard, 2005). When clinicians have limited signing skills, their efforts to engage signing deaf children can blunt their capacity to detect affective signals, thereby missing pertinent cues for emotional (Hindley et al., 1993) and other disorders. Even more experienced clinicians may misjudge a deaf child's linguistic capacities in either signed or spoken language, particularly during the first interview (e.g., when dealing with children with cochlear implants). For those cases, it is preferable to engage a professional sign language interpreter, ideally with experience in children's mental health (van Gent, 2000; Hindley & van Gent, 2002). Aspects of communication, content of the interview, procedure, and cooperation with the interviewer must be discussed both before and after the interview (van Gent, 2000; Hindley & van Gent, 2002). Most important, the interpreter will have eye contact with the child and may pick up subtle emotional cues (Turner, Klein, & Kitson, 2000), which may help the clinician to assess the nature of any problems. In general, the coexistence of deafness and psychiatric disorder can lead clinicians to an unwarranted assumption that deafness explains all—the phenomenon of "diagnostic shadowing" (Kitson & Thacker, 2000), a pitfall that also confounds the assessment and treatment of children with other handicapping conditions (Volkmar & Dykens, 2002). A diagnostic family interview is essential in dealing with deaf children and their families, as well as with hearing children in families with deaf parents or deaf siblings, perhaps even more so than with all-hearing families. As a rule, vital information on interactions, involvement, and intimacy and on the impact of communication within the family can thus be obtained.

Psychiatric evaluation may be difficult when deafness is combined with an intellectual disability. For deaf individuals with a profound disability, it may be wise to consider other communicative strategies, including the use of caregivers as interpreters of communication, and careful observation of behavior in different contexts (Carvill, 2001). In all such cases, a multi-informant approach to assessment, including reports from parents, teachers, and others, and significant data on background history are essential (van Gent et al., 2007). Differential diagnostic problems may be especially difficult to obtain in children and young people with combined hearing and visual impairments. One should always be quite sure that a visual disorder can be ruled out in children and adolescents with a hearing loss. One should take particular care not to miss sensory impairments when a complex, multicausal neuropsychiatric syndrome is combined with serious communicative problems. More frequently than in the examination or treatment of a deaf child, the clinician will encounter a need for more assistive resources, which may be hard to distinguish from abnormal psychological dependency.

PSYCHOLOGICAL TESTING

Psychological information based on test scores of cognitive, neuropsychological, academic, linguistic, and other aspects of functioning, personality, and psychopathology is one of the keystones of the multiaxial and multi-informant psychiatric assessment process as a whole (Rutter & Taylor, 2002). Caution should be employed when conducting psychological assessments of deaf children because most of these have been validated exclusively in hearing populations (also see *cognitive development* in chapter 10). Tests standardized or specifically developed for use with deaf people are still few in number, and many frequently used tests demand relatively high levels of intellectual and communicative abilities. Several studies (Blennerhassett, 2000; Orr, De Matteo, Heller, Lee, & Nguyen, 1987; Pollard, 2002; Maller & Braden, 2011) provide thorough accounts of the psychological assessment of deaf children. Carrying out psychological tests on hearing impairment demands a thorough knowledge of many domains, including the medical and audiological aspects of deafness and hearing impairment; the influence of deafness and other background variables (e.g., parental hearing status, educational placement, additional physical health problems) on development; cultural aspects of deafness; sociocultural differences between deaf and hearing people; differences within the heterogeneous population of deaf people; and the ability to estimate a child's level of communication and skills in various means of communication (e.g., signing, written language, speech, speechreading). In addition, good communication skills in various modalities are required. In everyday practice in specialized mental health settings, psychological assessments may take about twice as long with deaf children as with their hearing peers. This is partly because of the child's communication needs and partly because examiners need more time to be sure of the validity of their findings (Boer & van Gent, 1996).

AUTISM AND RELATED DISORDERS

Studies of deaf children attending audiology clinics found that autism and related disorders are more common in those youngsters than in hearing children. A diagnosis of autism was found in 5.3% of children with a moderate to profound hearing impairment (Jure, Rapin, & Tuchman, 1991). In another study 3.5% of autistic children was found to have a moderate to profound hearing loss (Rosenhall, Nordin, Sandström, Ahlsen, & Gillberg, 1999). In the latter study, intellectual impairment did not account completely for the higher incidence. One of the assumed causes of an increased prevalence of autism in deaf children is brain damage (van Gent, 2000; Hindley & van Gent, 2002). For instance, several studies have suggested that both deafness and autism spectrum disorder may be markers of brain damage in children with congenital rubella (Chess, 1977), cytomegalovirus (Steinlin, Nadal, Eich, Martin, & Boltshauser, 1996; Yamashita, Fujimoto, Nakajima, Isagai, & Matsuishi, 2003), or CHARGE association (Johansson et al., 2006) as a consequence of interference with prenatal central nervous-system development. A link between prenatal viral infections without interference with central nervous-system development and autism spectrum disorders is controversial (van Gent et al., 1997).

    The age of diagnosis of autism spectrum disorder is frequently later in deaf children than in hearing children (Juré et al., 1991; Roper, Arnold, & Monteiro, 2003), in part reflecting diagnostic shadowing (mentioned earlier). Equally important, early diagnosis of autism spectrum disorder in deaf children is complicated by the combined presence of communicative problems as a consequence of deafness and the restricted social involvement and frequently occurring atypical sensory responses (Rogers & Ozonoff, 2005) as a consequence of autism spectrum disorder. The basic impairments associated with autism are qualitatively different from those seen in other deaf children. Absent or otherwise abnormal involvement with the social world may distinguish autistic deaf children and adolescents from nonautistic deaf children with or without concomitant cognitive impairment (Rogers & Ozonoff, 2005). Social impairments may include deficient contacts with adults and peers, disordered social imitation, impaired joint attention, problems using eye gaze to regulate social interaction, and impaired social reciprocity. Other symptoms associated with abnormal joint attention include a failure to look at people, a lack of social smiling, and a lack of pointing (i.e., pointing would indicate an interest in objects) (Vig & Jedrysek, 1999). A preference for the world of objects and physical attributes (Rogers & Ozonoff, 2005) and impaired imaginative play in children of appropriate mental age may also be of differential diagnostic value. However, stereotypes or abnormal response to sensory stimuli may show considerable overlap between autism and mental retardation (Vig & Jedrysek, 1999), blindness (Jan, Freeman, & Scott, 1977) or serious deprivation (O'Connor et al., 2000).

Nevertheless, poor language skills stemming from deafness may be associated with delayed but not with impaired imaginative play (Hindley & van Gent, 2002). Unusual communication patterns and passivity without a discrepant social delay may be common in deaf children with intellectual impairment who are not autistic, and even clinicians with good signing skills can have difficulty detecting language disorder in sign language (ibid). Some autistic deaf children show significant improvement in social functioning when educated in signing environments (Jure et al., 1991; Roberts & Hindley, 1999). This suggests that the use of eye gaze as defined by the rules of signed languages is emotionally less confusing than the much more ambiguous and thus possibly distressing social eye gaze (see Woll in Hindley, 2000). Indeed, a body of research suggests an abnormal face-processing ability in children with autism spectrum disorder, including reduced attention or a lack of interest in the face and an aversion to the eyes (for an overview see Denmark, 2011). General face-processing impairment was not found in signing deaf children with autistic spectrum disorder (as compared to nonautistic signing deaf controls), suggesting that experience with observing faces for communication purposes during development may compensate for the autistic tendency to avoid looking at faces (ibid.). With signing autistic children, deficits in processing specific emotional expressions on the face were found, while no impairments in linguistic facial expressions were found, with the exception of a deficit in processing adverbials. These findings suggest a selective impairment in face processing in signing deaf children with autistic spectrum disorder for emotions that require attributions of emotional meaning and the mental state of others (ibid.).

The diagnosis of autism may be very complicated in children with a dual sensory impairment, especially when they also have an additional cognitive impairment. More than 60% of deaf-blind people have been found to have IQs lower than 50 in a nationwide survey in the United States (Klein Jensema, 1980), indicating that serious intellectual disability may often complicate the clinical picture with deaf-blind children and young people. Self-destructive behavior and other impulse-control disorders may be a symptom of an autism spectrum disorder, a mood or anxiety disorder, or a psychosis, but such problem behavior may also point to severe social deprivation and unmet communicative needs, which warrant specialist training in communication and social skills tailored to the socioemotional and communicative levels of the individual child. In a study of deaf-blind children with a profound intellectual disability (Hoevenaars-van den Boom, Anthonissen,

Knoors, & Vervloed, 2009), all of the deaf-blind participants showed social, communicative, and language impairment. Autistic participants with deaf-blindness demonstrated significantly more impairment in social reciprocity, in social initiatives, and in the use of communicative signals and functions. No differences were found in stereotyped behavior, quality of play, exploration, and problem-solving strategies.

BEHAVIORAL DISORDERS

Overrepresentation of children and adolescents with attention deficit or disruptive behavior disorders among those referred to clinics may reflect referral patterns (van Gent, 2000; Hindley & van Gent, 2002). Interestingly, a number of factors may explain a gradual decline in the higher incidence of behavioral disorder over a period of 15 years as observed among deaf children and adolescents referred to the national Dutch in- and outpatient mental health service (van Gent, Goedhart, & Treffers, 2012). First, the most urgent cases may have been dealt with in the first years of a new specialist service. Second, the development of special diagnostic and therapeutic intervention programs and consultation services may have had a positive effect on local expertise. Third, increased recognition of special communicative needs and the quality of communication with deaf children and adolescents may have contributed to the decline in referrals (Sinkkonen, 1994).

Attention deficit disorder (Kelly, Forney, Parker-Fischer, & Jones, 1993) and disruptive behavior may be associated with brain pathology, which occur in some types of deafness. A longitudinal study of children affected by congenital rubella (Chess, Korn, & Fernandez, 1971; Chess & Fernandez, 1980) found that early impulsiveness in those with deafness alone disappeared as the children acquired language and self-control skills. By contrast, impulsiveness persisted in deaf children with additional impairments. Oppositional behavior can be an expression of underlying feelings of impotence, anxiety, or sadness or an expression of frustration with communication difficulties (van Gent, 2000; Kelly et al., 1993). Symptoms of distractibility and overactivity may reflect a distracting visual environment or poor language matching in the classroom, leading to boredom (Hindley & Kroll, 1998) or undetected intellectual development, language impairment, or the side effects of drugs (Kelly et al., 1993). In a study of younger children (< 5 years of age), deaf children exhibited more oral language, sustained attention, and behavioral problems than did hearing controls (Barker et al., 2009). Language delay appeared to be both directly and indirectly associated with behavioral problems through an effect on attention (ibid.).

Finally, positively biased self-perceptions in the social domain have been associated with behavioral disorders in deaf adolescents, as in hearing peers (van Gent, Goedhart, & Treffers, 2011). Theoretically, this could reflect the impact of younger mental age and lower level of sociocognitive maturity in a number of young deaf people, as has been found in hearing peers (ibid.; Harter, 2006; van Gent, Goedhart, Knoors, Westenberg, & Treffers, 2012).

EMOTIONAL DISORDERS

Studies using a combination of parent and teacher questionnaires and diagnostic interviews (Hindley et al., 1994; van Gent et al., 2007), as well as parent (van Eldik et al., 2004) and self-reports (van Eldik, 2005; Cornes et al., 2006) all found that rates of both emotional and behavioral problems are greater in deaf children and adolescent populations than in hearing age peers groups. In representative samples of school-attending children with a moderate to profound hearing loss (Fellinger et al., 2009) and deaf adolescents (van Gent et al., 2007) with normal IQ, emotional disorders were found to be more prevalent than behavioral disorder refuting the idea that deaf children and young people are more likely to display more behavioral than emotional problems. The risk of emotional disorder increases in children and adolescents who are rejected (van Gent et al., 2011), teased, isolated, or maltreated (Fellinger et al., 2009) as reported by others, but causal relations have to be studied further. A modest correlation has been found between the probability of being bullied, isolated, or maltreated and the ability to make oneself understood (ibid.). Emotional problems may also be missed because poor signing skills may prevent hearing parents, teachers, and professionals from recognizing emotional problems, anxiety, or a mood disturbance (Hindley & van Gent, 2002). As in hearing peers, emotional disorders in deaf adolescents are better detected during personal interviews (Hindley et al., 1994; van Gent et al., 2007). Evidence suggests that a lesser degree of deafness, an acquired or syndromal cause or the presence of additional neurological disorder may be regarded as stress inducing deafness related circumstances which moderate the association between low global self-esteem and emotional disorder (van Gent et al., 2011). For instance, a profitable use of residual hearing may make it more difficult to accept deafness (Polat, 2003). Deaf young people with more profitable hearing may be challenged more intensively than deaf peers with less profitable hearing to cope with social-communicative values and customs in the hearing oriented world, and perceive their limited skills in spoken language as an "incorrigible" personal shortcoming (van Gent et al., 2011). Secondly, deaf children with an acquired or syndromal cause have to cope more often with physical restrictions, handicap and its interpersonal consequences, compared to deaf people with an uncomplicated genetic cause and no history of neurological or other disorder (ibid). Moreover,, social isolation—being deaf in a large majority of hearing peers—may be an independent, chronic, interpersonal risk factor for emotional disorder (i.e., irrespective of the level of global self-esteem) (van Gent, 2012). The display of emotion used to illustrate narratives in sign language must not be confused with an affective disorder. The latter is pervasive and persistent, whereas the former changes rapidly and is congruent with the narrative (Roberts & Hindley, 1999). Behavioral problems that have distinct beginnings and endings, with no clear response to changes in circumstances, may derive from depression (Kitson & Thacker, 2000).

SCHIZOPHRENIA AND OTHER PSYCHOSES

Psychotic disorders are not more common in young people who are deaf than in hearing adolescents (Kitson & Thacker, 2000). Because the syntax of sign language is very different from that of spoken language, disorders of thinking can be misattributed (Evans & Elliott, 1987; Jenkins & Chess, 1996). Equally, accurate assessments of thought disorder and abnormal experiences can be difficult to obtain (Kitson & Thacker, 2000). Nevertheless, phenomena such as clang associations and flight of ideas have been clearly identified in deaf adults with psychotic disorders (ibid.). Visual or somatic hallucinations are observed more often in deaf patients with schizophrenia (i.e., in about 50% of cases) than in hearing patients (i.e., in about 15% [visual] or 5% [somatic] of cases) (Cutting, 1985). Contrary to expectations, auditory hallucinations, some of which are verbal, do occur in deaf patients with schizophrenia (Du Feu & McKenna, 1999). In addition, a distinction can be made between subvisual voice imagery and true visual hallucinations; deaf individuals who report seeing an image of a voice may in fact experience a visual percept of voice articulations (Atkinson, 2006; Atkinson, Gleeson, Cromwell, & O'Rourke, 2007). In line with the subvocal thought hypothesis (Frith & Done, 1988), the perception of voices may be the result of failing to recognize one's own subvocal thoughts and instead perceiving them as having an external locus of control (Atkinson et al., 2007). Moreover, it is possible that the perceptual characteristics of voice hallucinations closely reflect the variety of experience of real-life communication, language, and sound among deaf individuals (ibid.). Profoundly deaf individuals without auditory memory may experience seeing an image of a voice signing or lips moving in their mind. But patients with experience and memory of hearing speech, either due to acquired deafness or the profitable use of residual hearing, may describe voices in auditory terms. Moreover, patients with severe language deprivation and impoverished acquisition of speech or sign language may be incapable of experiencing either auditory characteristics or perception of subvisual imagery of voice articulation (Atkinson, 2006; Atkinson et al., 2007).

SPECIAL GROUPS OF CHILDREN

Children with Otitis Media with Effusion

Otitis media with effusion (OME) can lead to transient, sometimes severe, conductive hearing impairment. Although earlier reports suggested that this could result in long-lasting impaired language skills and behavioral difficulties (Chalmers, Stewart, Silva, & Mulvena, 1989), more current studies now indicate that fluctuating hearing impairment that is experienced with OME causes serious formal language difficulties less often (Bennett & Haggard, 1999), with transient delays in speech, language, and academic skills, (Roberts, Burchinal, & Zeisel, 2002). In addition, OME and accompanying symptoms may lead to communication problems, altered social responses, emotional distress (including mood and anxiety problems), irritability, and other behavioral problems such as difficulties with attention and activity, as well as sleep and balance problems (Brouwer et al., 2005). Temporary or recurrent hearing loss may be especially distressing to young children who have an already existing hearing impairment of another etiology, as they may feel particularly anxious about losing their residual hearing and may not be capable of articulating what is happening.

Hearing Children of Deaf Parents

More than 90% of deaf parents have hearing children (Singleton & Tittle, 2000). Knowledge of the development of hearing children of deaf parents is relatively limited (Meadow-Orlans, 1995; Singleton & Tittle, 2000). These studies, as well as a comprehensive anthropological study of 150 grown children of signing deaf parents (Preston, 1994), indicate that most deaf parents are generally competent and caring but do experience the stress of being deaf in a hearing world (Singleton & Tittle, 2000).

Hearing children of deaf parents are often mediators between the deaf and the hearing culture. Although the use of sign language is a central component of being deaf and often a source of pride, some deaf people see their sign language as less valued than spoken language; they may be concerned about the adequacy of the signed linguistic environment for their hearing child (ibid.). This may lead some to choose not to sign with their hearing child and to rely on inadequate spoken language (ibid.). In other circumstances, hearing children are drawn into the role of communicator/interpreter for their parents. Some of them see these experiences as adverse inasmuch as they "parentify" the child at an early age; others, however, find that these experiences lead to "greater adaptiveness, resourcefulness, curiosity and 'worldliness'" (ibid., p. 228).

Deaf parents may have difficulty in accessing information about parenting, and their own childhood within a hearing family may not have provided them with good models of parenting. This may cause them to feel insecure or incompetent as parents (ibid.). In some respects, the experience of deaf parents of hearing children can be compared to that of parents who are raising children of ethnic backgrounds different from their own (ibid.).

Most of the grown-up hearing children of deaf parents studied by Preston (1994) acknowledged some difficulties in their childhood but attributed these as much to the hearing society's response to their parents as to their parent's "failings." Their roles as interpreters and advocates were linked to experiences that were both fulfilling and hurtful. In a similar vein many described a sense of divided loyalty toward their deaf parents and their hearing grandparents.

Little is known about the psychological well-being of hearing children of deaf parents, but perhaps a characteristic pattern should not be expected (Hindley & van Gent, 2002). Clinical experience in specialist services suggests that emotional difficulties and family problems are relatively common. In a survey of referrals to the Dutch national mental health service for deaf and hard of hearing children and their families (van Gent, Goedhart, & Treffers, 2012), hearing children of one or two parents with a hearing impairment appeared to grow up much more often in a one-parent family than comparable referrals of hearing children of hearing parents. Referral reasons for hearing children of parents with a hearing impairment tended more frequently to mention emotional disorder and less frequently to cite behavioral, autistic spectrum, or some other disorder than appears to be the case for referrals of hearing children of hearing parents. Hypothetically, this could partly reflect higher distress among these children, but whether this also applies to nonreferred children is not known.

Children with Cochlear Implants

Effects of cochlear implantation (CI) may vary considerably among children and adolescents. In general, the beneficial effects of CI are most marked in the least adverse communicative circumstances (e.g., low background noise, simultaneous group conversations, joining and maintaining interaction in larger groups; Bat-Chava & Deignan, 2001; Martin, Bat-Chava, Lalwani, & Waltzman, 2010; Punch & Hyde, 2011). There are still few studies on the longer-term effects of CI on psychosocial development. In a longitudinal Swedish study (Tvingstedt, & Ahlström, 2002; Tvingstedt & Preisler, 2006), children with a cochlear implant reported a positive appreciation of their implant, but they and their parents shared the awareness that they are still deaf. Overall, studies indicate that language ability irrespective of modality is an important predictor of psychosocial well-being (Dammeyer, 2009). In one study (Bat-Chava, Martin, & Kosciw, 2004), children with cochlear implants demonstrated a faster improvement in social skills following the development of communication skills over time than children with conventional hearing aids. Whether this reflects an improvement in the forming of a mental perspective, as has been suggested by the authors and others (Remmel & Peters, 2009), remains a subject for further research. Compared with hearing children, delays in theory of mind development were reported for both deaf children with CI and with conventional hearing aids (Peterson, 2006; Wellman, Fang, & Peterson, 2011).

No differences in executive functions were found between children with and without a cochlear implant (Figueras, Edwards, & Langdon, 2008; Hintermair, Schenk, & Sarimski, 2011) despite the finding of a positive association between language ability and executive functioning in one of these studies (Figueras et al., 2008). From a perspective based on a combination of current cultural values and empirical findings, a bilingual approach to the education of most deaf children is still advocated (Petitto & Holowka, 2002; Marschark, 2007; Preisler, 2007). However, at least in industrialized countries, a growing number of children who have received a cochlear implant early on have an opportunity to learn a spoken language, and spoken language will become a first language for many of them (Knoors & Marschark, 2012). At the same time, sign language will likely remain important not only for other children and adults but also for younger children with a CI and their parents, for whom it can serve as both an adjunct to spoken language and an effective bridge before and after implantation (ibid.). Research variations notwithstanding, CI has definitively changed the face of deafness (Marschark, 2007).

So far, findings on the effect of CI on self-concept are rather inconsistent (Martin, Bat-Chava, Lalwani, & Waltzman, 2010; Leigh, Maxwell-McCaw, Bat-Chava, & Christiansen, 2009; Nicolas & Geers, 2003; Schorr, Fox, & Roth, 2006), as are reports about psychosocial problems from parents, teachers, or the implantees themselves (Dammeyer, 2009; Edwards, Kahn, Broxholme, & Langdon,, 2006; Fellinger et al., 2009; Huber & Kipman, 2011; Knutson, Ehlers, Wald, & Tyler, 2000a, 2000b; Leigh et al., 2009). Differences in study design, measures, informants, and composition of samples hamper comparisons across studies. No effect of CI on psychiatric diagnosis was observed in a population-based study with children and adolescents (6–16 years of age), using diagnostic parental interviews and parental and teachers' questionnaires (Fellinger et al., 2009). In another population-based study, the degree of hearing loss and CI use were unrelated to the increased level of self-reported depression in children with a hearing impairment (Theunissen et al., 2011). In a more recent publication on the same study sample, lower levels of anxiety and other, both internalizing and externalizing, symptoms were reported in children with a CI than in children with a hearing aid (Theunissen, 2013). These findings should be interpreted with caution, however, inasmuch as failure to control for additional variables (e.g., gender, age of onset of deafness, co-occurring disabilities, socioeconomic status) may lead to an overestimation of the effectiveness of CI (Stacey, Fortnum, Barton, & Summerfield, 2006). Failure to control for other variables (e.g., average hearing level, age) (ibid.) or shorter use of CI (Figueras et al., 2008) may lead to an underestimation. Thus, more research on psychological development and the prevalence of mental health problems in well-described homogeneous samples of children with and without a CI is much needed. Cochlear implantation has definitively changed the face of deafness (Marschark, 2007).

Intervention

Systematic clinical and scientific interest in mental health problems in deaf people began around 1950. Probably the earliest psychiatric study of deaf individuals was done by Hansen in 1929, who reported that deaf adults were overrepresented in psychiatric hospitals and that the average duration of stay was significantly longer than that of hearing patients (Vernon & Daigle-King, 1999). In 1955, the first specialist mental health clinic for deaf adults opened in the United States, and in 1972 Schlesinger and Meadow opened the first ambulatory treatment service for deaf children in the United States (Vernon, 1980). While these initial mental health services for deaf adults (Rainer & Altschuler, 1966) and children (Vernon, 1980; Schlesinger and Meadow, 1972) were being established in North America, similar interest was developing in northern Europe (van Gent, 2012). Though mental health services for deaf children and adolescents are better developed in Western European countries and the United States than elsewhere, these facilities are still inadequate. As exemplified by the special-interest group for deaf children and families of the European Society for Mental Health and Deafness, the foundation of international networks of professionals promotes an exchange of information, resources, and experience among practitioners, thus creating an international platform for cooperation and support in this low-incidence, highly specialized area of care. Most services emphasize the importance of the sociocultural model of deafness, consultation with both the Deaf community and parents of children with a hearing impairment, and a mixed team of deaf and hearing professionals, in which the latter are expected to achieve high levels of sign language proficiency.

After an initial assessment of the children, the same range of outpatient and inpatient treatments should be provided as for hearing children and their families. Treatment often has to be organized nearer to the child's home because of the distance to the specialized service. Because of their scarcity, specialized services are often provided by consultants to local clinics or ambulatory services (van Gent, 1999).

Evans and Elliott (1987) describe specific pitfalls in both the psychotherapy of deaf and hard of hearing children and the value of deaf therapists. Interpreters in family and group therapy may increase the complexity of transference relationships (Hoyt, Siegelman, & Schlesinger, 1981). Medication may produce side effects, such as extrapyramidal consequences and sedation, which impede communication because they influence visual alertness, motor function, and coordination, and thus the skills needed for signing, speechreading, speaking, and writing (Sleeboom-van Raaij, 1997). Also, children with a hearing impairment may be unable to adequately explain the effects and side effects of the medication prescribed (Hindley & van Gent, 2002), and the brains of children with cognitive impairments may also place them at greater risk of these effects. Because of the increased occurrence of physical comorbidity, contraindications must be taken into careful consideration.

Specialist or Generic Services

Specialist services for deaf children do not fit neatly into existing models of services, but the fundamental characteristic of services to this population involves the communication and visual-spatial aspects of orientation (Hindley & van Gent, 2002). Basically, referral of deaf children to specialized mental health services should be guided by the visual-spatial and communication needs of the child and the complexity of the case. Where specialist services are unavailable, clinicians should seek additional resources (e.g., sign language interpreters) and be prepared to use nonverbal means of communication (ibid.).

ADULT OUTCOME OF DEAFNESS

The findings of a study of the deaf population in upper Austria (Fellinger et al., 2005) suggest that deaf adults are more likely to experience higher levels of mental and/or physical distress and poorer quality of life than hearing adults in the general population. In the domain of social relationships, adults who were hard of hearing were found to have less satisfying social relationships than deaf individuals who used sign language (Fellinger, Holzinger, Gerich, & Goldberg, 2007). In a Norwegian survey, deaf adults were found to have more symptoms of anxiety and depression than hearing individuals (Kvam, Loeb, & Tambs, 2006). A community survey of deaf adults (Checinski, 1993) has suggested an increased rate of psychiatric disorder, with perhaps a third of adults experiencing an episode of depression more frequently than hearing adults. In London, referrals for depression and anxiety disorder have grown in relation to improvements in service provision (Kitson & Thacker, 2000). In line with the clinical experience with adolescents, greater drug use (Austen & Checinski, 2000) and abuse (Vernon & Daigle-King, 1999) among deaf adults have been reported. In a hospital in Massachusetts, fewer psychotic disorders and more posttraumatic stress, as well as developmental, mood, anxiety, and personality disorders, were found among the deaf inpatients than among the hearing inpatients (Black & Glickman, 2006). Because so few specialized deaf inpatient units exist, they serve a much broader range of clients than do regular units, including patients with dangerous and violent behavior, serious social skills deficits, and language disfluency related to longstanding language deprivation.

Evaluating 13 years of ambulatory mental health care for adults with a hearing impairment, De Bruin & De Graaf (2005) note that to date the majority of adult referrals to their service are deaf. They conclude that specialist mental health services should promote specialist services for clients who have a postlingual, partial, or progressive hearing impairment, as this subgroup is quite likely to experience high rates of mental health problems, partly due to the difficulty of losing one's hearing and having to accept this condition without having the support of a socio-cultural group to identify with, such as the signing Deaf community.

CONCLUSIONS

Chapters 10 and 11

Our knowledge of the developmental pathways of deaf children continues to grow. Until recently, the main psychological focus has been on the effects of deafness and hearing loss on key developmental experiences and on the effects of society's response to sensory deficits. The growing body of studies on physical, environmental, deafness-related, and intrapersonal risk factors that may help to identify a more specific focus for preventive, diagnostic, and treatment interventions for subgroups of deaf people is encouraging. Currently, governmental initiatives to ban educational discrimination and to promote the integration of deaf children and others, the development of early newborn hearing screening and intervention programs, the introduction of CI, and insights from neuroscience and developmental psychology have a great impact on the challenges faced by deaf children and their parents, who sometimes struggle to deal with life in two worlds and attempt not to get stuck somewhere in between them (Marschark, 2007). To date, in most developed countries specialized mental health services for deaf children and their families are underrepresented. As assessment and treatment needs for the deaf population and their families are still underserved (Leigh & Pollard, 2011; van Gent, 2012), the main goal for service planning should be to improve the accessibility and the quality of both kinds of services—for deaf as well as hard of hearing people. In general, regular health and mental health professionals should be aware of the specific character of many mental health needs of deaf people and the differences between deaf and hearing people in social, cultural, cognitive, and other psychological domains. They should also be cognizant of the fact that deafness and hearing loss may be viewed as a cultural difference by many and as a disability by others, depending on the background and focus of the deaf individuals and their families or the perception of the professionals or caregivers who seek to help these children. An integrated approach to mental health issues and research will continue to be crucial.

REFERENCES

Aplin, D. Y. (1985). Social and emotional adjustments of hearing-impaired children in special schools. *Journal of the British Association of Teachers of the Deaf, 9,* 84–94.

Aplin, D. Y. (1987). Social and emotional adjustments of hearing-impaired children in ordinary and special schools. *Educational Research Volume, 29,* 56–64.

Arnold, P., & Atkins, J. (1991). The social and emotional adjustment of primary hearing-impaired children integrated in primary schools. *Educational Research, 33,* 223–228.

Atkinson, J. R. (2006). The perceptual characteristics of voice hallucinations in deaf people: Insights into the nature of subvocal thought and sensory feedback loops. *Schizophrenia Bulletin, 32,* 701–708.

Atkinson, J. R., Gleeson, K., Cromwell, J., & O'Rourke, S. (2007). Exploring the perceptual characteristics of voice hallucinations in deaf people. *Cognitive Neuropsychiatry, 12*(4), 339–361.

Austen, S., & Checinski, K. (2000). Addictive behavior and deafness. In P. Hindley & N. Kitson (Eds.), *Mental health and deafness* (pp. 232–252). London: Whurr.

Barker, D. H., Quittner, A. L., Fink, N. E., Eisenberg, L. S., Tobey, E. A., Niparko, J. K., & the CDaCI Investigative Team. (2009). Predicting behavior problems in deaf and hearing children: The influences of language, attention, and parent-child communication. *Development and Psychopathology, 21,* 373–392.

Bat-Chava, Y., & Deignan, E. (2001). Peer relations of children with cochlear implants. *Journal of Deaf Studies and Deaf Education, 6,* 186–199.

Bat-Chava, Y., Martin, D., & Kosciw, J. G. (2004). Longitudinal improvements in communication and socialization of deaf children with cochlear implants and hearing aids: Evidence from parental reports. *Journal of Child Psychology and Psychiatry, 46,* 1287–1296.

Beck, G., & de Jong, E. (1990). *Opgroeien in een Horende Wereld.* [Growing up in a hearing world]. Twello, the Netherlands: Van Tricht.

Bennett, K. E., & Haggard, M. P. (1999). Behavior and cognitive outcomes from middle ear disease. *Archives of Disease in Childhood, 80,* 28–35.

Black, P. A., & Glickman, N. S. (2006). Demographics, psychiatric diagnoses, and other characteristics of North American deaf and hard-of-hearing inpatients. *Journal of Deaf Studies and Deaf Education, 11,* 303–321.

Blennerhassett, L. (2000). Psychological assessments. In P. Hindley & N. Kitson (Eds.), *Mental health and deafness* (pp. 185–205). London: Whurr.

Boer, F., & van Gent, T. (1996). Evaluatie 1993 1994 1995 *Afdeling voor doven en ernstig slechthorenden de Vlier. Intern evaluatierapport Academisch Centrum Kinder- en Jeugdpsychiatrie Curium.* Oegsteest: Curium (Evaluation 1993 1994 1995 Department for deaf and severely hard of hearing children and adolescents de Vlier. Internal evaluation report Academic Center Child and Adolescent Psychiatry Curium. Oegstgeest: Curium).

Brouwer, C. N. M., Maillé, A. R., Rovers, M. M., Grobbee, D. E., Sanders, E. A. M., & Schilder, A. G. M. (2005). Health-related quality of life in children with otitis media. *International Journal of Pediatric Otorhinolaryngology, 69,* 1031–1041.

Carvill, S. (2001). Sensory impairments, intellectual disability and psychiatry. *Journal of Intellectual Disability Research, 45,* 467–483.

Chalmers, D., Stewart, I., Silva, P., & Mulvena, A. (1989). *Otitis media with effusion in children: The Dunedin study.* Clinics in Developmental Medicine, 108. London: MacKeith Press.

Checinski, K. (1993). *An estimate of the point prevalence of psychiatric disorder in prelingually deaf adults living in the community.* MD thesis, Cambridge University.

Chess, S. (1977). Follow-up report on autism in congenital rubella. *Journal of Autism and Childhood Schizophrenia, 7,* 69–81.

Chess, S., & Fernandez, P. (1980). Do deaf children have a typical personality? *Journal of the American Academy of Child Psychiatry, 19,* 654–664.

Chess, S., Korn, S. J., & Fernandez, P. B. (1971). *Psychiatric disorders of children with congenital rubella.* New York: Brunner & Mazel.

Conrad, R. (1979). *The Deaf Schoolchild.* Harper & Row Ltd, London.

Cornes, A., Rohan, M. J., Napier, J., & Del Rey, J. M. (2006). Reading the signs: Impact of signed versus written questionnaires on the prevalence of psychopathology among deaf adolescents. *Australian & New Zealand Journal of Psychiatry, 40,* 665–673.

Cutting, J. (1985). *The psychology of schizophrenia.* London: Churchill Livingstone.

Dammeyer, J. (2009). Psychosocial development in a Danish population of children with cochlear implants and deaf and hard-of-hearing children. *Journal of Deaf Studies and Deaf Education, 15,* 50–58.

De Bruin, E., & De Graaf, R. (2005). What do we know about deaf clients after 13 years of community mental health? An analysis of the PsyDoN database from 1987 to 1999. *American Annals of the Deaf, 149,* 384–393.

Denmark, T. (2011). *Do deaf children with autism spectrum disorder show deficits in the comprehension and production of emotional and linguistic facial expressions in British Sign Language?* PhD dissertation, University College, London.

Du Feu, M., & McKenna, P. J. (1999). Prelingually profoundly deaf schizophrenic patients who hear voices: A phenomenological analysis. *Acta Psychiatrica Scandinavica, 99,* 453–459.

Edwards, L., Kahn, S., Broxholme, C., & Langdon, D. (2006). Exploration of the cognitive and behavioural consequences of paediatric cochlear implantation. *Cochlear Implants International, 7,* 61–76.

Evans, J. W., & Elliott, H. (1987). The mental status examination. In H. Elliott, L. Glass, & J. W. Evans (Eds.), *Mental health assessment of deaf clients: A practical manual* (pp. 83–92). San Diego: Little, Brown.

Fellinger, J., Holzinger, D., Dobner, U., Gerich, J., Lehner R., Lenz, G., & Goldberg, D. (2005). Mental distress and quality of life in a deaf population. *Journal of Social Psychiatry and Psychiatric Epidemiology, 40,* 737–742.

Fellinger, J., Holzinger, D., Gerich, J., & Goldberg, D. (2007). Mental distress and quality of life in the hard of hearing. *Acta Psychiatrica Scandinavica, 115,* 243–245.

Fellinger, J., Holzinger, D., Sattel, H., Laucht, M., & Goldberg, D. (2009). Correlates of mental health disorders among children with hearing impairments. *Developmental Medicine & Child Neurology, 51,* 635–641.

Figueras, B., Edwards, L., & Langdon, D. (2008). Executive function and language in deaf children. *Journal of Deaf Studies and Deaf Education, 13,* 362–377.

Freeman, R. D., Malkin, S. F., & Hastings, J. O. (1975). Psychological problems of deaf children and their families: A comparative study. *American Annals of the Deaf, 120,* 275–304.

Frith, C. D., & Done, D. J. (1988). Towards a neuropsychology of schizophrenia. *British Journal of Psychiatry, 153,* 437–443.

Fundudis, T., Kolvin, I., & Garside, R. (1979). *Speech retarded and deaf children: Their psychological development.* London: Academic Press.

Goodman, R. (1997). The Strength and Difficulties Questionnaire: A research note. *Journal of Child Psychology and Psychiatry, 38,* 581–586.

Harter, S. (2006). Self-processes and developmental psychopathology. In D. Cicchieti & D. J. Cohen (Eds.), *Developmental psychopathology* (pp. 370–418). Hoboken, NJ: Wiley.

Hindley, P. A. (1997). Psychiatric aspects of hearing impairments. *Journal of Child Psychology and Psychiatry, 38,* 101–117.

Hindley, P. A. (2000). Child and adolescent psychiatry. In P. Hindley & N. Kitson (Eds.), *Mental health and deafness* (pp. 42–74). London: Whurr.

Hindley, P. A., Hill, P. D., & Bond, D. (1993). Interviewing deaf children, the interviewer effect: A research note. *Journal of Child Psychology and Psychiatry, 34,* 1461–1467.

Hindley, P. A., Hill, P. D., McGuigan, S., & Kitson, N. (1994). Psychiatric disorder in deaf and hearing impaired children and young people: A prevalence study. *Journal of Child Psychology and Psychiatry, 35,* 917–934.

Hindley, P. A., & Kroll, L. (1998). Theoretical and epidemiological aspects of attention deficit and overactivity in deaf children. *Journal of Deaf Studies and Deaf Education, 3,* 64–72.

Hindley, P., & van Gent, T. (2002). Psychiatric aspects of specific hearing impairments. In M. Rutter & E. Taylor (Eds.), *Child and adolescent psychiatry* (4th ed.) (pp. 842–857). Oxford: Blackwell Science.

Hintermair, M. (2007). Prevalence of socioemotional problems in deaf and hard of hearing children in Germany. *American Annals of the Deaf, 152,* 320–330.

Hintermair, M., Schenk, A., & Sarimski, K. (2011). Executive Funktionen, kommunikative Kompetenz und Verhaltensauffälligkeiten bei hörgeschädigten Kindern: Eine explorative Studie mit Schülern einer schulischen Einrichtung für Hörgeschädigte [Executive functioning, communicative competence and behavior disorders in deaf and hard-of-hearing students]. *Empirische Sonderpädagogik, 2,* 83–104.

Hoevenaars-van den Boom, M. A. A., Anthonissen, A. C. F. M., Knoors, H., & Vervloed, M. P. J. (2009). Differentiating characteristics of deafblindness and autism in people with congenital deafblindness and profound intellectual disability. *Journal of Intellectual Disability Research, 53,* 548–558.

Hoyt, M. F., Siegelman, E. Y., & Schlesinger, H. S. (1981). Special issues regarding psychotherapy with the deaf. *American Journal of Psychiatry, 138,* 807–811.

Huber, M., & Kipman, U. (2011). The mental health of deaf adolescents with cochlear implants compared to their hearing peers. *International Journal of Audiology, 50,* 146–154.

Jan, J. E., Freeman, R. D., & Scott, E. P. (1977). *Visual impairment in children and adolescents.* New York: Grune & Stratton.

Jenkins, I. R., & Chess, S. (1996). Psychiatric evaluation of perceptually impaired children: Hearing and visual impairments. In M. Lewis (Ed.), *Child and adolescent psychiatry: A comprehensive textbook* (2nd ed.) (pp. 526–534). Baltimore: Williams & Wilkins.

Johansson, M., Råstam, M., Billstedt, E., Danielsson, S., Strömland, K., Miller, M., & Gillberg, C. (2006). Autism spectrum disorders and underlying brain pathology in CHARGE association. *Developmental Medicine & Child Neurology, 48,* 40–50.

Jure, R., Rapin, I., & Tuchman, R. F. (1991). Hearing impaired autistic children. *Developmental Medicine and Child Neurology, 33,* 1062–1072.

Kammerer, E. (1988). *Kinderpsychiatrische Aspekte der schweren Hörschädigung* [Child psychiatric aspects of severe hearing impairment]. Stuttgart: Ferdinand Enke.

Kelly, D., Forney, J., Parker-Fischer, S., & Jones, M. (1993). The challenge of attention deficit disorder in children who are deaf or hard of hearing. *American Annals of the Deaf, 138,* 343–348.

Kitson, N., & Thacker, A. (2000). Adult psychiatry. In P. Hindley & N. Kitson (Eds.), *Mental health and deafness* (pp. 75–98). London: Whurr.

Klein Jensema, C. (1980). A profile of deaf-blind children with various types of educational facilities. *American Annals of the Deaf, 125,* 896–900.

Knoors, H., & Marschark, M. (2012). Language planning for the 21st century: Revisiting bilingual language policy for deaf children. *Journal of Deaf Studies and Deaf Education.* doi: 10.1093/deafed/ens018

Knutson, J. F., Ehlers, S. L., Wald, R. L., & Tyler, R. S. (2000a). Psychological consequences of pediatric cochlear implant use. *Annals of Otology, Rhinology, and Laryngology, 109,* 109–111.

Knutson, J. F., Ehlers, S. L., Wald, R. L., & Tyler, R. S. (2000b). Psychological predictors of pediatric cochlear implant use and benefit. *Annals of Otology, Rhinology, and Laryngology, 109,* 100–103.

Kouwenberg, M., Rieffe, C., Theunissen, S. C. P. M., & Rooij, M. de (2012). Peer victimization experienced by children and adolescents who are deaf or hard of hearing. *PLoS ONE* 7:e52174. DOI:10.1371/journal.pone.0052174.

Kvam, M., H., Loeb, M., & Tambs, K. (2006). Mental health in deaf adults: Symptoms of anxiety and depression among hearing and deaf individuals. *Journal of Deaf Studies and Deaf Education, 12*, 1–7.

Leigh, I. W., Maxwell-McCaw, D., Bat-Chava, Y., & Christiansen, J. B. (2009). Correlates of psychosocial adjustment in deaf adolescents with and without cochlear implants: A preliminary investigation. *Journal of Deaf Studies and Deaf Education, 14*, 244–259.

Leigh, I. W., & Pollard, R. Q. (2011). Mental health and deaf adults. In M. Marschark & P. E. Spencer (Eds.), *The Oxford handbook of deaf studies, language, and education, Vol. 1* (pp. 214–226). Oxford: Oxford University Press.

Loots, G., & Devisé, I. (2003). The use of visual-tactile communication strategies by deaf and hearing fathers and mothers of deaf infants. *Journal of Deaf Studies and Deaf Education, 8*, 31–42.

Maller, S. J. (2003). Intellectual assessment of deaf people: A critical review of core concepts and issues. In M. Marschark & P. E. Spencer (Eds.), *Deaf studies, language, and education* (pp. 415–463). Oxford: Oxford University Press.

Maller, S. J., & Braden, J. T. (2011). Intellectual assessment of deaf people: A critical review. In M. Marschark & P. E. Spencer (Eds.), *The Oxford book of deaf studies, language and education* (vol. 2, pp. 473–485). New York: Oxford University Press.

Marschark, M. (2007). *Raising and educating a deaf child* (2nd ed.). Oxford: Oxford University Press.

Martin, D., Bat-Chava, Y., Lalwani, A., & Waltzman, S. B. (2010). Peer relationships of deaf children with cochlear implants: Predictors of peer entry and peer interaction success. *Journal of Deaf Studies and Deaf Education, 16*, 108–120.

Mathos, K. K., & Broussard, E. R. (2005). Outlining the concerns of children who have hearing loss and their families. *Journal of the American Academy of Child and Adolescent Psychiatry, 44*, 96–100.

Meadow-Orlans, K. (1995). Parenting with a sensory or physical disability. In M. Borstein (Ed.), *Handbook of parenting: Vol. 4. Applied and practical considerations* (pp. 57–84). Hillsdale, NJ: Erlbaum.

Mitchell, T. V., & Quittner, A. L. (1996). A multimethod study of attention and behavior problems in hearing-impaired children. *Journal of Clinical Child Psychology, 25*, 83–96.

Nicolas, J. G., & Geers, A. E. (2003). Personal, social, and family adjustment in school-aged children with a cochlear implant. *Ear & Hearing, 24*, 69S–81S.

O'Connor, T. G., Rutter, M., Beckett, C., Keaveney, L., & Kreppner, J. M., and the English and Romanian Adoptees Study Team (2000). The effects of global severe privation on cognitive competence: Extension and longitudinal follow-up. *Child Development, 71*, 376–390.

Orr, F. C., De Matteo, A., Heller, B., Lee, M., & Nguyen, M. (1987). Psychological assessment. In H. Elliott, L. Glass, & J. W. Evans (Eds.), *Mental health assessment of deaf clients: A practical manual*, pp. 94–142. Boston: Little, Brown.

Peterson, C. C. (2006). Theory-of-mind development in oral deaf children with cochlear implants or conventional hearing aids. *Journal of Child Psychiatry, 45*, 1069–1106.

Petitto, L. A., & Holowka, S. (2002). Evaluating attributions of delay and confusion in young bilinguals: Special insights from infants acquiring a signed and spoken language. *Sign Language Studies, 3*, 4–33.

Pollard, R. (2002). Ethical conduct in research involving deaf people. In V. Gutman (Ed.), *Ethics in mental health and deafness* (pp. 162–178). Washington, DC: Gallaudet University Press.

Polat, F. (2003). Factors affecting psychosocial adjustment of deaf students. *Journal of Deaf Studies and Deaf Education, 8*, 325–339.

Preisler, G. (2007, September 11–14). *Will learning from the past give us insight for the future concerning the psychosocial development of deaf children with cochlear implants?* Plenary presentation at the Seventh European Congress on Mental Health and Deafness, "Joining Forces," Haarlem, the Netherlands.

Preisler, G., Tvingstedt, A. L., & Ahlström, M. (2002). The development of communication and language in deaf preschool children with cochlear implants. *Child: Care, Health and Development, 28,* 403–418.

Preston, P. (1994). *Mother Father Deaf.* Cambridge, MA: Harvard University Press.

Punch, R., & Hyde, M. (2011). Social participation of children and adolescents with cochlear implants: A qualitative analysis of parent, teacher, an child interviews. *Journal of Deaf Studies and Deaf Education, 16,* 474–493.

Rainer, J. D., & Altschuler, K. Z. (1966). *Comprehensive mental health services for the deaf.* New York: New York State Psychiatric Institute, Department of Medical Genetics.

Remmel, E., & Peters, K. (2009). Theory of mind and language in children with cochlear implants. *Journal of Deaf Studies and Deaf Education, 14,* 218–236.

Roberts, C., & Hindley, P. (1999). Practitioner review: The assessment and treatment of deaf children with psychiatric disorders. *Journal of Child Psychology and Psychiatry, 40,* 151–167.

Roberts, J. E., Burchinal, M. R., & Zeisel, S. A. (2002). Otitis media in early childhood in relation to children's school-age language and academic skills. *Pediatrics, 110,* 1–11.

Rogers, S. J., & Ozonoff, S. (2005). Annotation: What do we know about sensory dysfunction in autism? A critical review of the empirical evidence. *Journal of Child Psychology and Psychiatry, 46,* 1255–1268.

Roper, L., Arnold, P., & Monteiro, B. (2003). Co-occurrence of autism and deafness: Diagnostic considerations. *Autism, 7,* 245–254.

Rosenhall, U., Nordin, V., Sandström, M., Ahlsen, G., & Gillberg, C. (1999). Autism and hearing loss. *Journal of Autism and Developmental Disorders, 29,* 349–357.

Rutter, M., Graham, P., & Yule, W. (1970). *A neuropsychiatric study in childhood.* Clinics in Developmental Medicine 35/36. London: Spastics International Medical Publications.

Rutter, M., & Taylor, E. (2002). Clinical assessment and diagnostic formulation. In M. Rutter & E. Taylor (Eds.), *Child and adolescent psychiatry* (4th ed.) (pp. 18–31). London: Blackwell.

Schlesinger, H. S., & Meadow, K. P. (1972). *Sound and sign: Childhood deafness and mental health.* Berkeley: University of California Press.

Schorr, E. A., Fox, N. A., & Roth, F. P. (2006). Research report to parents on social and emotional functioning of children with cochlear implants. College Park: University of Maryland at College Park.

Singleton, J. L., & Tittle, M. D. (2000). Deaf parents and their hearing children. *Journal of Deaf Studies and Deaf Education, 5,* 221–236.

Sinkkonen, J. (1994). *Hearing impairment, communication, and personality development.* Unpublished doctoral dissertation, University of Helsinki.

Sleeboom-van Raaij, I. (1997). *Psycho-pharmacological treatment and deafness: Hazards and highlights.* Presentation at the Fourth International Congress of the European Society for Mental Health and Deafness, Manchester.

Smith, P. K., & Sharp, S. (1994). *School bullying: Insights and perspectives.* London: Routledge.

Spronk-van Hal, C. M. (1994). Research into psychological instruments for deaf children and adolescents. In A. Karacostas (Ed.), *Deafness and well-being: Contributions of deaf and hearing professionals to the improvement of mental health and deafness practice.* Proceedings of the Third International Congress, European Society for Mental Health and Deafness, UNESCO Headquarters, December 14–16. Paris: ESMHD.

Stacey, P. C., Fortnum, H. M., Barton, G. R., & Summerfield, A. Q. (2006). Hearing-impaired children in the United Kingdom, I: Auditory performance, communication skills, educational achievements, quality of life, and cochlear implantation. *Ear & Hearing, 27*, 161–186.

Steinlin, M. I., Nadal, D., Eich, G. F., Martin, E., & Boltshauser, E. J. (1996). Late intrauterine cytomegalovirus infection: clinical and neuroimaging findings. *Pediatric Neurology, 15*, 249–253.

Sullivan, P., Brookhouser, P., & Scanlan, M. (2000). Maltreatment of deaf and hard of hearing children. In P. Hindley & N. Kitson (Eds.), *Mental health and deafness* (pp. 148–184). London: Whurr.

Theunissen, S. C. P. M. (2013). *Psychopathology in hearing impaired children.* Doctoral dissertation, Leiden University. Leiden: Gildeprint, Enschedé.

Theunissen, S. C. P. M., Rieffe, C., Kouwenberg, M., Soede, W., Briaire, J. J., & Frijns, J. H. M. (2011). Depression in hearing-impaired children. *International Journal of Pediatric Otorhinolaryngology, 75*, 1313–1317.

Turner, J., Klein, H., & Kitson, N. (2000). Interpreters in mental health settings. In P. Hindley & N. Kitson (Eds.), *Mental health and deafness* (pp. 297–310). London: Whurr.

Tvingstedt, A. L., & Preisler, G. (2006). *A psychosocial follow-up study of children with cochlear implants in different school settings.* EDUCARE. Malmö: Holmbergs.

van Eldik, T. (2005). Mental health problems of Dutch youth with hearing loss as shown on the youth self-report. *American Annals of the Deaf, 150*, 11–16.

van Eldik, T., Treffers, P. D. A., Veerman, J. W., & Verhulst, F. C. (2004). Mental health problems of deaf Dutch children as indicated by parents' responses to the Child Behavior Checklist. *American Annals of the Deaf, 148*, 390–395.

van Gent, T. (1999*). Factors complicating psychiatric assessment and treatment of deaf and severely hard of hearing children.* Plenary presentation at the First European Symposium on Deaf Children and Mental Health of the ESMHD. Children and Families Special Interest Group. National Deaf Services, Pathfinder Mental Health Services, NH, Danbury, UK.

van Gent, T. (2000). Onderzoek en diagnostiek bij dove kinderen en jeugdigen [Assessment and diagnosis in deaf children and youth]. In F. C. Verhulst & F. Verheij (Eds.), *Kinder- en jeugdpsychiatrie: Onderzoek en diagnostiek [Child and adolescent psychiatry: Assessment und diagnosis]* (pp. 393–407). Assen, the Netherlands: Van Gorcum.

van Gent, T. (2012). *Mental health problems in deaf and severely hard of hearing children and adolescents: Findings on prevalence, pathogenesis, and clinical complexities and implications for prevention, diagnosis, and intervention.* Doctoral dissertation, Leiden University, Leiden. Leiden: Mostert.

van Gent, T., Goedhart, A. W., Hindley, P. A., & Treffers, P. D. A. (2007). Prevalence and correlates of psychopathology in a sample of deaf adolescents. *Journal of Child Psychology and Psychiatry, 48*, 950–958.

van Gent, T., Goedhart, A., Knoors, H., Westenberg, P. M., & Treffers, P. D. A. (2012, February 20). Self-concept and ego development in deaf adolescents: Associations with social context and deafness-related variables, and a comparison with hearing adolescents. *Journal of Deaf Studies and Deaf Education*, doi: 10.1093/deafed/ens002

van Gent, T., Goedhart, A. W., & Treffers, P. D. A. (2011). Self-concept and psychopathology in deaf adolescents: Preliminary support for moderating effects of deafness-related characteristics and peer problems. *Journal of Child Psychology and Psychiatry, 52*, 720–728.

van Gent, T., Goedhart, A. W., & Treffers, P. D. A. (2012). Characteristics of children and adolescents in the Dutch national in- and outpatient mental health service for deaf and hard of hearing youth over a period of 15 years. *Research in developmental Disabilities, 33*, 1333–1342.

van Gent, T., Heijnen, C., & Treffers, P. D. A. (1997). Autism and the immune system. *Journal of Child Psychology and Psychiatry, 38,* 337–349.

Verloes, A. (2005). Updated diagnostic criteria for CHARGE syndrome: A proposal. *American Journal of Medical Genetics, 133A,* 306–308.

Vernon, M. (1968/2005). Fifty years of research on the intelligence of deaf and hard-of-hearing children: A review of literature and discussion of implications. *Journal of Rehabilitation of the Deaf, 1,* 1–12. Reprinted in the *Journal of Deaf Studies and Deaf Education, 10,* 225–231.

Vernon, M. (1980). Perspectives on deafness and mental health. *Journal of Rehabilitation of the Deaf, 13,* 8–14.

Vernon, M., & Daigle-King, B. (1999). Historical overview of inpatient care of mental patients who are deaf. *American Annals of the Deaf, 144,* 51–61.

Vig, S., & Jedrysek, E. (1999). Autistic features in young children with significant cognitive impairment: Autism or mental retardation? *Journal of Autism and Developmental Disorders, 29,* 235–248.

Volkmar, F. R., & Dykens, E. (2002). Mental retardation. In M. Rutter & E. Taylor (Eds.), *Child and adolescent psychiatry* (4th ed.) (pp. 697–710). Oxford: Blackwell.

Vostanis, P., Hayes, M., Du Feu, M., & Warren, J. (1997). Detection of behavioural and emotional problems in deaf children and adolescents: Comparison of two rating scales. *Child: Care, Health and Development, 23,* 233–246.

Wellman, H. M., Fang, F., & Peterson, C. C. (2011). Sequential progressions in a theory-of-mind scale: Longitudinal perspectives. *Child Development, 82,* 780–792.

Yamashita, Y., Fujimoto, C., Nakajima, E., Isagai, T., & Matsuishi, T. (2003). Possible association between congenital cytomegalovirus infection and autistic disorder. *Journal of Autism and Developmental Disorders, 33,* 455–459.

.

12

The Mother-Child Relationship and Language Development Disorders: Studies of Deaf Adolescent Children of Hearing Parents

Joanna Kobosko

Relative to the language competence of their hearing peers from hearing families and their deaf peers from Deaf families, the vast majority (about 70%) of deaf children of hearing parents tend to have substandard language competence in either spoken or natural sign language (e.g., Black & Glickman, 2006; Fellinger et al., 2005; Glickman, 2007; Kitson & Fry, 1990; Krakowiak, 2003; Punch & Hyde, 2011; Scheetz, 2004). Most deaf adolescent sign language users or sign-supported-system users employ some form of "pigeon sign language" (Wojda, 2009, 2010), which is usually insufficient or inadequate.

It should be remembered that deafness per se and "being deaf does not, in itself, predetermine a given child's path of development any more than does the fact of being left-handed or being six-feet tall. Rather, the context in which deafness occurs, and the interpretations placed on it by others, will be far more influential in shaping the child's future progress and adjustment" (Koster & Meadow-Orlans, 1991, p. 300).

It is worth noting that although language development in deaf adolescents is related to their psychological functioning, there is no comparable DSM-IV category for simple language retardation in hearing children. Interestingly, in a study of deaf and hard of hearing children and adolescents, using the Semistructured Clinical Interview for Children and Adolescents (SCICA), the rate of diagnosable mental disorders was found to correlate positively with the level of language deprivation and mode of communication (van Gent, Goedhart, Hindley, & Treffers, 2007). This state of affairs is the result of persistent ineffectiveness of medical, linguistic, psychological, and educational interventions facilitating language development in

193

deaf children and adolescents, suggesting that we need to seek new solutions. Perhaps if we were to adopt the interpersonal perspective (Stern, 1985, 1995; Zalewska, 1998a), which means considering the quality of the mother-child relationship and its effects on developmental disorders, including the language development of hearing-intact children and those with a hearing impairment, we would be able to suggest new directions of clinical theory and practice in this field.

RESEARCH DIRECTIONS AND INTERVENTIONS IN THE FIELD OF LANGUAGE DEVELOPMENT AND DEPRIVATION IN DEAF CHILDREN AND ADOLESCENTS FROM HEARING FAMILIES: IMPLICATIONS FOR THE MOTHER (PARENT)/ CHILD RELATIONSHIP

In many European countries the question of how to facilitate language development in children with a hearing impairment who have hearing-intact parents is conceptualized in terms of intervention: medical, linguistic, educational, and psychological. Since hearing parents of children with a hearing impairment typically choose the language or method of communication to be used with their children, the child's development and the parent-child relationship may be affected by a number of psychological issues.

Medical Intervention from the Point of View of the Deaf Child's Language Development and the Mother-Child Relationship

Typically, medical intervention is oriented toward the development of spoken language, auditory communication, or visual-auditory communication. To that end, hearing aids or cochlear implants (CIs), as well as hearing and speech therapy, are often utilized. Given that cochlear implants have traditionally been (and still are?) viewed as a sign of parents' denial of their child's deafness (e.g., Hindley, 2000), deaf children with cochlear implants should theoretically have considerable difficulty with their psycholinguistic development because denial of deafness would negatively affect the mother-child relationship. Studies of the deaf population with implants in the United States between 1972 and 2000 found that about 30% communicated by means of spoken language and lived in the hearing community, 30% communicated by means of natural sign language and were a subculture of the Deaf community, and about 30% were "in between," neither here nor there, identified with neither of these communities, and did not achieve satisfactory mastery of either spoken language or natural sign language (Bat-Chava & Deignan, 2001).

From the point of view of linguistic functioning, this deaf population with CIs in-cludes individuals who are proficient in spoken language and/or natural sign lan-guage. Therefore, these findings indirectly suggest, among other things, that we must consider other aspects (or mechanisms) of the mother-child relationship that enable the deaf child to acquire either spoken language or natural sign language. Cochlear implantation increasingly offered to deaf infants under 1 year of age may have other functions (e.g., ones that facilitate the mother-child relationship) and are not necessarily indicators of denial of the child's deafness.

Studies of reading comprehension, an ability related to language develop-ment, in deaf secondary-school graduates have shown that these children achieve a level that does not exceed the primary school grade-four level for hearing chil-dren (Allen, 1986; Kroese, Lotz, et al., 1986; DiFrancesca, 1972; after Spencer, Barker, & Tomblin, 2003). They have also shown that about 30% of deaf children are classified as functional illiterates (Traxler, 2000; after Spencer et al., 2003). As far as reading with comprehension is concerned, a similar pattern can be ob-served in deaf children and adolescents with CIs: Compared with hearing peers, pupils with cochlear implants exhibited reading levels that became increasingly delayed with age. The older the deaf pupils, the greater their delay in reading in comparison to their hearing peers. For example, a delay of 3 years was found in deaf 11–13-year-old pupils and 4–5 years in these same pupils when they were 15–17 years of age (Thoutenhoofd, 2006; after Marschark, Rothen, & Fabich, 2007). Other researchers found that 50% of deaf 18-year-old CI users read below the primary school grade-four equivalent for hearing pupils, and 50% of this group exceeded the primary school grade-four level for hearing pupils (Traxler, 2000; after Marschark, Rothen, & Fabich, 2007). An Australian study of communica-tion, psychosocial, and educational outcomes of children and adolescents with cochlear implants (CI before age 18) found that "70% of the children were judged by their teachers to be below the median level of the class in academic achieve-ments, particularly in literacy and numeracy" (Punch & Hyde, 2011, p. 7).

The research findings on development of spoken language in deaf adolescents with cochlear implants suggest that although these adolescents quite often achieve clarity of spoken language, they lack the refined, complex language necessary to understand school curricula (Archbold, 2005; after Marschark, Rothen, & Fabich, 2007) and also reveal deficient narrative-building skills, including poor grammar, impoverished vocabulary, use of shorter sentences, less complex sentences, wrong verb conjugation, and numerous other language errors (e.g., Crosson & Geers, 2001; after Marschark, Rothen, & Fabich, 2007; Gacek, 2007; Klatter-Folmer, Kolen, van Hout, & Verhoeven, 2006; Spencer et al., 2003). These researchers conclude that there are still some deficits in expressive (spoken) language for this group.

With regard to literacy, the numerous studies of language development in deaf adolescents with CIs allow one to conclude that, although these young peo-ple's language skills are much more advanced than those of adolescents using conventional hearing aids, they are still significantly inferior to those of their hearing peers. Whatever the type of hearing prosthesis, deaf adolescents also have less-than-adequate narrative competence, which also causes concern if we look at this fact from an interpersonal perspective. Which elements of the mother-child relationship could be causing these delays in language development in deaf adolescents from hearing families? Given the hypothesis that maternal distress interrupts self-narration (Ricoeur, 1990/2005), are the narrative difficulties that are apparently manifested in (both spoken and natural sign) language related in any way to difficulties in the relationship between mothers and their deaf children? If so, then deaf adolescents cannot "tell themselves by themselves," and this also finds expression in their multiple language disfluencies.

Linguistic Intervention from the Point of View of the Deaf Child's Language Development and the Mother-Child Relationship

In linguistic intervention, optimization of language development in deaf children of hearing parents involves choosing the best language for the deaf child. According to psychologists or psychiatrists representing the cultural model of deafness (e.g., Schlesinger & Meadow, 1972; Glickman, 1996), the best choice would be manual language, given its natural visibility to the deaf child. Hence advocates of this linguistic option believe that hearing parents of deaf children should learn to use and/or support a natural sign language or bilingual option. However, it is important to remember that a hearing mother's choice of this approach does not automatically ensure a good relationship with her child (e.g., Kamińska, 2003). Given that some deaf people living in hearing families become highly competent users of spoken or/and sign language, it follows, from application of the interpersonal approach, that the development of language competence in deaf children is dependent on shared qualities of the mother-child relationship.

This reasoning is confirmed by research findings on the various properties of the interaction between the hearing mother and the deaf child. A British study (Janjua, Woll, & Kyle, 2002) has found that the quality of the interaction between hearing mothers and (about 3-year-old) deaf children was independent of communication mode, provided that the level of language proficiency, assessed with the Bristol Language Development Scales, used to assess both sign and spoken language development, was comparable. Another study (Wallis, Musselman, and McKay, 2004) has drawn attention to another dimension of mother-child interaction: early mode match (either auditory/oral or sign match) in early childhood and its effect on language development and mental health. In this study the auditory/oral group consisted of children who used spoken English both in early childhood and in adolescence, as did their mothers. Children who used manual language both in early childhood (prior to 5 years of age) and adolescence, as did their mothers, constituted the sign match group. The sign mismatch group consisted of children who used sign in adolescence but not in early childhood or who, although signing in early childhood, had a mother who did not. The researchers found a significant positive effect of good match on the mental functioning of deaf adolescents from hearing families regardless of whether spoken or natural sign language was used. To assess the deaf adolescents' mental functioning (symptoms of psychopathology), the Youth Self-Report (YSR), developed by Achenbach and then modified by the investigators (see Wallis, Musselman, & McKay, 2004), was applied. Deaf, sign-mismatched adolescents' mental functioning was significantly inferior to that of sign- or oral-matched adolescents.

Observations of language development in deaf children in an experimental bilingual class (Bouvet, 1982/1996) and deaf children with cochlear implants in a bilingual program in Sweden (Preissler, 2007) suggest that bilingualism is a viable approach: The greater the deaf children's mastery of spoken language, the more competent they were in natural sign language, and vice versa. When viewed in the context of the quality of the (hearing) mother–(deaf) child relationship, this finding also suggests the existence of shared qualities that facilitate the deaf child's language development, no matter what language is being learned.

Psychological Intervention, Language Development in Deaf Children, and Mother-Child Relations

Early intervention programs typically offered to hearing mothers with deaf children involve psychoeducation and are based on the assumption that the difference in hearing status has a negative effect on mother-child interactions (e.g., Marschark & Spencer, 2003; Hindley, 2000): The mother can hear, whereas her child cannot; therefore the mother needs to be provided with a choice of model interaction formats. These will basically take the form of either hearing mother–hearing child or deaf mother–deaf child interaction models, with the dominant modality being auditory in the former and visual/tactile (that is, natural sign language) in the latter (Koester, Brooks, & Traci, 2000). This approach to language development ignores the relationship between language development and the mother-child relationship. In other words, no attention is paid to how the mother experiences her own motherhood and her child's deafness, as well as the processes embedded in this experience, such as mourning the loss of the normal, healthy and hearing-intact child (Zalewska, 1998a, 1998b).

Though each of these approaches has the goal of facilitating optimal speech and language development and functioning of the deaf child (and the child's family), more attention needs to be paid to the interpersonal approach, which argues that the child's language development is closely associated with the development of maternal identity in the child's mother and the quality of mother-child relations (Stern, 1985, 1995).

AUDIOLOGICAL (TRADITIONAL) AND INTERPERSONAL APPROACH TO HEARING MOTHER–DEAF CHILD RELATIONSHIP AND THE CHILD'S LANGUAGE DEVELOPMENT

When a hearing mother learns that her child is deaf, her psychological reaction is usually complex. Three aspects of this reaction have been identified: trauma, loss (the mother mourns the loss of her child, who was healthy and had typical hearing), and verbal impairment in her relations with her child (Zalewska, 1998a, 1998b). While the first two might be present for reasons other than the child's deafness, the experience of verbal impairment has a unique impact on the mother–deaf child experience: impairment of her capacity to "be with" her child, as well as the triggering of a mourning process, in which the mother experiences the loss of her "healthy," "normal," or "hearing" child. This process affects the quality of her relationship with her child.

In many countries early intervention programs for families with deaf children are based largely on an educational or "rehabilitative" approach with the deaf child's mother. Mothers are usually expected to develop a strategy or style that will facilitate mother-child interactions focused on language development (as mentioned earlier; see the section on linguistic intervention from the point of view of the deaf child's language development and the mother-child relationship).

Representatives of the interpersonal approach, including Daniel Stern (1985, 1995) in the United States and Marina Zalewska (1998a, 1998b) in Poland, suggest that the quality of the mother-child relationship affects the child's psychological growth, including language development. Linguistically accessible childhood experiences are those that have become part of the child's social self and are shared with and named by the mothers; the active mechanism for this mother-child interaction is emotional attunement. The efficiency of this mechanism partly depends on the mother's psychological condition and her capacity to experience emotional and psychological states (Stern, 1985, 1995) and hence on the properties of her inchoate representation of her child and her relations with the child. The repressed self is deprived of language's organizing functions (Stern, 1985).

When the (hearing) mother hears the audiological diagnosis, her mental representation of her (deaf) child is suddenly reorganized, and hearing and speech now occupy a central place in this representation. Parental activity is now action oriented (rather than experience oriented). The parents want the child to learn to hear and speak so that the child can "live a normal life." We know this not only from the clinical experience of psychologists who work with deaf children's parents but also from a British study (Young & Tattersall, 2007) of parents of very young deaf children diagnosed at 25 weeks of age on the average within the framework of a screening program for newborn babies and infants. When the child is diagnosed as deaf, the mother's representation very soon begins to include motifs such as "hearing, speech, and language" or "normal speech and the chance to be like hearing children," and the "deficit and disease" model of deafness begins to prevail. Parents also typically feel that something can be done to "cure their child of deafness," a pattern also identified in parents of children who have cancer. There is no room for a deaf child in this early, altered representation. We learn from this report that the mother has very little capacity for emotional attunement with her child, which according to Stern (1985) constitutes affective mechanism present in a mother-child relationship. Young and Tatersall (2007) identified four categories of parental representations of their very young deaf child. These representations were oriented toward the following: (a) normal development (10 parents), (b) avoidance of developmental pathology (8 parents), (c) no fantasies concerning the child's development (7 parents), and (d) giving support and ensuring the use of a variety of ways to communicate with the child regardless of whether spoken or natural sign language is used (2 parents). These results show that, at the level of representation analysis, the vast majority of hearing parents of very young deaf children need professional assistance to develop their relationships with their deaf offspring. Hearing mothers' representations of their deaf children are therefore clearly focused on the deafness but also contain a change motif, and the majority of descriptive categories involve the child's external attributes (Zalewska, 1998a).

Much information about representations of the mother-child relationship can also be gleaned from numerous studies of interactions between hearing mothers and their deaf children. These studies have found, for example, a typically controlling and directive interaction style, greater insensitivity to the child's communications, maternal intrusiveness, negative emotions, or interaction ruptures due to errors and misunderstandings. A review of this work is presented elsewhere (cf. Kobosko & Zalewska, 2011). Furthermore, the greater the language delay in the deaf child of hearing parents, the more likely it is that the mother-child interactions will be rated as dysfunctional and the child as "difficult" (Pipp-Siegel, Sedey, & Yoshinaga-Itano, 2002).

To summarize, mothers' difficulties in experiencing themselves as mothers of deaf children and the mechanisms these difficulties trigger or modify (e.g., verbal impairment, emotional attunement, verbalization of emotions), as well as the consequent specific quality of the mother-child relationship, may significantly contribute to severe language deprivation in deaf adolescents of hearing parents. We must not forget, however, that there are also mothers whose relations with their children facilitate the development of speech and language, whether spoken or natural sign language (as already mentioned), and achievement of satisfactory language competence in deaf adolescents.

The present analysis of the link between the quality of the mother-child relationship and language deprivation in the child is derived from the proposition formulated by Zalewska (1998a) on the basis of her clinical experience: Poor language skills are related to a disturbed development of the sense of self in the child (both deaf and hearing) and by the mother's difficulty in experiencing herself as her child's mother. More and more research is focusing on the psychological state of the mother and the child, for example, more frequent depression (Kushalnagar et al., 2007; Kobosko & Kosmalowa, 2000) and its effect on the psychological development of the deaf child.

THE PROJECT

The research project presented in this chapter is part of a larger study of the maternal identity of hearing mothers of deaf adolescents and the personal identities of the adolescents themselves (Kobosko, 2007). The study discussed here focused on the effects of the mother-child relationship on the development of personal identity in deaf adolescents and its possible contribution to the adolescents' language delay. The following issues are addressed:

1. The impact of the emotional verbalization mechanism in the (hearing) mother– (deaf) child relationship on the adolescent's experience of self-as-deaf (when the adolescent uses either spoken language or natural sign language).
2. The impact of shared mother-father emotions in the (hearing) mother-father relationship (the emotion verbalization mechanism) on the adolescent's experience of self-as-deaf (the emotion verbalization mechanism) when the adolescent uses either spoken language or natural sign language.
3. The hearing mother's experience of self-as-mother-of-adolescent-deaf-child (metaphors) as related to the child's deafness and the use or nonuse of spoken and/or natural sign language.

Participants

The participants were prelingually deaf adolescents aged 18–22 years ($n = 41$), including 10 competent users of spoken language, 10 competent users of natural sign language, 11 less competent users of spoken and natural sign language, 10 very incompetent users of spoken and natural sign language, and their hearing mothers. The audiological criterion of deafness was a hearing level of 90 dB or more in the better ear. Only transcribed interviews ("What is it like to be deaf?") with deaf adolescents with high levels of competence in spoken language or natural sign language were submitted to narrative analysis. The remaining deaf adolescents, whose spoken or natural sign language competence was limited, were not analyzed in this part of the study (i.e., narrative analysis). The control group consisted of 40 hearing adolescents and their hearing mothers.

Method

Semistructured interviews about self-experience were conducted with the hearing mothers as well as their deaf and hearing children. Interviews with the mother focused on the topic of motherhood. Mothers' responses to selected interview questions (e.g., "How's [son's/daughter's first name] been doing lately?" and then "How are you experiencing this situation?") were used to assess the mothers' representations of their relationships with their children as well as with their children's fathers (e.g., "Motherhood involves the fact that the child has a father. How did your relationship with [son's/daughter's first name] father look initially?" or "When deafness was diagnosed in your son/daughter, was this an important moment in your relationship?"). The interview material was transcribed, and selected fragments were submitted to narrative analysis. The maternal representations of their relationships with their children and with their children's fathers were used to make inferences about the affective properties of these representations (narrative analysis and verbalization of emotions; discussed later in this section), including maternal emotions shared with the child's father.

Interviews with the deaf adolescents (having high language competence in either spoken or natural sign language) centered around the topic of "What's it like to be deaf?" Those with the hearing children focused on "What's it like to be a person who has a deficit?" A native sign language user was used with the deaf adolescents using natural sign language (per the bi-bi model; see Napier & Cornes, 2003). The interview material was transcribed, and selected fragments were submitted to narrative analysis.

Narrative analysis was used to describe the emotion verbalizations of the mothers and the adolescents. Five levels of verbalization, ranging from "no verbalization of emotions" to "verbalization of a variety of emotions, both positive and negative," were suggested. These criteria are a modification of those adopted by Lane and Schwartz in their Levels of Emotional Awareness Scale (LEAS) (Novick-Kline, Turk, Mennin, Hoyt, & Gallagher, 2005; Szczygieł & Kolańczyk, 2000):

No verbalization of emotions: narratives in which emotional content is missing and/or action tendencies are verbalized (LEAS stages I and II)

Diffuse emotions: narratives in which mental states and feelings are verbalized in a generalized way without indicating any of the primary emotions specified by Lane and Schwarz (e.g., I feel anxious; I'm worried; I regret that . . .)

Positive emotions: narratives in which mental states and feelings are verbalized as positive emotions specified in the LEAS as primary emotions, such as joy (e.g., I'm happy; we love each other) or enjoyment (e.g., I like).

Negative emotions: narratives in which mental states and feelings are verbalized as negative emotions specified in the LEAS as primary emotions, such as fear, sadness, and anger (e.g., I'm overcome with sadness when I recall those moments; I'm afraid; I'm angry with him).

Positive and negative emotions (differentiated): narratives in which mental states and feelings are verbalized by distinguishing positive and negative emotions specified by the LEAS as primary, such as fear, sadness, anger, or joy (e.g., I'm sorry that Ania has to work so hard, but I'm glad when she gets a good grade on a test).

The narratives produced in response to selected items on the "motherhood" interview and "What's it like to be deaf?" / "What's it like to be a person who has a deficit?" were coded by expert judges. These methods were used to elicit descriptions of the aforementioned maternal representations of the mothers' relationships with their children and their children's fathers as well as the adolescents' self-representations of "self-as-deaf" or "self with a deficit" (hearing adolescents). Expert judges rated these representations on five dimensions of "verbalization of emotion" (yes/no). The hypotheses about relationships between maternal verbalization of emotions and adolescent verbalizations of emotions, taking the deaf/hearing dimension into consideration, were tested statistically by means of correspondence analysis.

RESULTS

Representation of the Mother/(Deaf) Child Relationship in Hearing Mothers and Adolescents' Experience of Self-as-Deaf

A significant relation was found between the way mothers experience their relationship with their adolescent offspring (deaf and hearing) and the way the adolescents experience their deafness vs. some other psychological or physical deficit (correspondence analysis: $\chi^2 (17) = 37.46$, p < 0.003).

Interview with Rafał's Mother

Interviewer: How's Rafał been doing lately? How are you experiencing this situation?

Rafał's mother: When I see, for example, that he's sitting lost in thought, I ask him, "What's happened? Is anything wrong? Tell Mum what's up. Mum will explain." I simply want to know what's on his mind. He doesn't always want to tell me about his problems. He sometimes says that there's nothing wrong, but I can see that he's engrossed in thought, that there's something . . . **I'm afraid** [boldface type indicates verbalization of negative emotions] just simply that he might break down at some point . . . I'm sure he knows that he's different from the others, you know, his hearing colleagues. Well, but he's never said that **he's resentful**. He's never asked why things are like they are.

Interview with Ania's Mother

Interviewer: How's Ania been doing lately? How are you experiencing this situation?

Ania's mother: Well, I try to cheer her up [and let her know] that in the end all will be well . . . I mean her studies and all that . . . I try to help her. I can't explain physics to her, but we sometimes go for consultations. And above all I support her, I support her psychologically, so to speak, but also materially . . . because I buy her all these books she asks me for . . . [no verbalization of emotion].

Hearing mothers of linguistically competent deaf adolescents using spoken or natural sign language revealed a number of difficulties in their relationships with their children. These mothers do not verbalize their experiences of or emotions, for example, regarding their child's deafness in their mother-child relationship (cf. interview with Ania's mother), or if they do verbalize them, they are negative (cf. interview with Rafał's mother). These mothers introduce negative emotions or experiences that are "hard to express" (secondary alexithymia; Kobosko, 2007) into their relationship with their deaf child. The difficulties the hearing mothers have in their relationship with their child coincide with problems that linguistically competent deaf adolescents have experiencing themselves as deaf (cf. interview with Alicja). It is worth adding that hearing mothers of hearing adolescents experience positive emotions in their relationships with their adolescent children.

Interview with Alicja

[Alicja says she has a "hearing impairment"; she communicates in spoken Polish.]

Interviewer: What did you feel when you found out that you have a hearing impairment?

Alicja: Well, I discovered that when I speak—I had this feeling that I'm different from other people. That I'm simply . . . I thought that everybody was the same. Then I just discovered that I was simply different.

Interviewer: What do you feel?

Alicja: **Disgust**. I mean, it's like being inferior . . . worthless. Well, I feel so—well, I feel that I'm disabled.

Maternal Representation of the Child's Father and Adolescents' Experience of Self-as-Deaf

We found that the mother's sharing of her emotions and experiences surrounding her relationship with the child's father (measured at the level of the mother's mental representation of the father) affects adolescents' experience of self-as-deaf (deaf adolescents) vs. self-as-psychologically or physically deficient (hearing adolescents) (correspondence analysis: χ^2 (25) = 47.03, p < 0.005). We also found that maternal sharing of emotions with the father of a linguistically proficient deaf adolescent coincides with lack of verbalization of emotion (i.e., in deaf adolescents, difficulty experiencing one's deafness).

Interview with Maciek's Mother

Interviewer: When Maciek was diagnosed as deaf was this an important moment in your [marital] relationship?

Maciek's mother: Well, altogether this was an absolute shock. It was the end of the world, so to speak. It was such a shock that, that, that one couldn't cope with it . . . Our friends' reactions, well, some of them withdrew immediately because it's better to . . . from such people because they have a problem . . . We didn't show it . . . **we**, so to speak, **suffered alone** [sharing emotions with the child's father].

Interview with Monika

[Monika calls herself a "deaf person"; she communicates in natural sign language.]

Interviewer: What did you feel when you discovered that you are deaf?

Monika: That I couldn't hear.

Interviewer: What did you feel?

Monika: That I speak and cannot hear, that I do not register sounds . . . Well, that's how I felt about it . . . now it's normal, no problem at all [no verbalization of emotion].

Representation of Self-as-Mother-of-a-Deaf-Child (Metaphors) and Speaking vs. Not Speaking in Deaf Adolescents

We also used metaphors in the interviews with mothers ("motherhood"). Unlike usual clinical practice, in which it is the clinician who uses metaphors as a form of intervention, each mother was asked to use a metaphor (comparison) in the form of "an image, word, or sentence" that comes to mind "now, when we have been talking for a while about the subject of [her] being a mother [of a deaf child], a comparison showing what [her] motherhood is like." People sometimes use metaphors consciously but view their meaning more symbolically (i.e., at an unconscious level) (Barker, 1997). This is the rationale behind the use of metaphoric communication in the clinical setting (ibid.). Also, both therapists and their clients/patients may be less reluctant to express and accept meanings that are communicated indirectly. Metaphorically expressed meanings are usually only partly accessible to reflection.

Maternal metaphors (i.e., communication of one's experience of self-as-mother-of-a-deaf-child) are very different in mothers of deaf adolescent "speakers," who are very proficient users of spoken (Table 1) or natural sign language (Table 2), and mothers of deaf adolescent "nonspeakers," who have very limited competence in spoken and natural sign language (Table 3).

Mothers of highly linguistically competent deaf children, whatever their language, tend to make references to "life, mental states, and emotions." They experience mothering a deaf child as, for example, "happiness"; "being proud of [herself] for having such a [daughter]"; "mental burden"; "great joy." Mothers of

TABLE 1.   Maternal Metaphors Used by Hearing Mothers of Deaf Adolescents
Who Are Very Proficient in Spoken Polish (All Names Changed)

Hearing Mothers of Deaf Adolescents with Proficiency in Spoken Language	Maternal Metaphors: Word, Image, or Sentence (Utterance Quotations)
mother of Wojtek (boy, age 21)	Well, I'm certainly never bored . . . Wojtek is one great mystery . . . nothing comes to mind.
mother of Bronek (boy, age 18)	Like a journey
mother of Diana (girl, age 18)	She's my little sun . . . joy . . . my joy
mother of Julia (girl, age 18)	Like a tempest just now. With lightning right now . . . But I think that someday . . . someday a mellow May afternoon with a rainbow will come, and I hope it comes soon.
mother of Marta (girl, age 18)	To be the mother of Marta . . . precisely this Marta . . . well, for me, well, really, is to be proud of myself that, that, that that's what she's like.
mother of Maciek (boy, age 18)	To be a mother of a deaf child is like . . . like walking against the wind
mother of Anna (girl, age 21)	To be moved, that's for certain. Great love, I feel only positive things; to be Ania's mother—pure joy of life
mother of Katarzyna (girl, age 19)	It's a great pleasure to be Kasia's mother.
mother of Mikołaj (boy, age 19)	An eternal problem . . . maybe not so awful, but a problem nevertheless; a great psychological burden. And I'm worried all the time.
mother of Alicja (girl, age 19)	It's satisfying to be Ala's mother. I'm very proud that I'm her mother.

"nonspeaking" deaf children tend to use metaphors that refer to the inanimate world; they experience mothering a deaf child as, for example, "like a chocolate box full of delicious chocolates"; "a huge, colorful umbrella, so huge that it almost covers . . . "; "I simply feel that I am a mother of a child. I'm at a loss for words." These metaphors may reflect "dead spaces" (lacunae) in their experience of self-as-mother-of-a-deaf-child.

TABLE 2. Maternal Metaphors Used by Hearing Mothers of Deaf Adolescents Who
Are Very Proficient in Natural Sign Language (All Names Changed)

Hearing Mothers of Deaf Adolescents with Proficiency in Natural Sign Language	Maternal Metaphors: Word, Image or Sentence (Utterance Quotations)
mother of Ewa (girl, age 19)	Well, I'm glad that . . . I have her. And I definitely wouldn't swap Ewa for . . . even for . . . five hearing children.
mother of Dorota (girl, age 19)	Well, she's been everything, simply everything to me, everything. Everything I had, I've poured into her, the children—all my love.
mother of Mateusz (boy, age 18)	Nothing, I think. No, I can't say. Nothing comes to mind . . .
mother of Małgosia (girl, age 19)	No, well, just . . . being Małgosia's mother is wonderful and beautiful. Yes, it's a challenge for me. And that seems to be it.
mother of Marysia (girl, age 19)	I'm so happy to have such a daughter. Really. I don't think I can express it any other way.
mother of Emilia (girl, age 19)	Fighting with windmills, powerlessness
mother of Monika (girl, age 19)	An undulating sea . . . perhaps . . . I've always been swimming, up, approaching—perhaps that, perhaps. I've tried—to find out so as, heaven forbid, not to ignore, neglect. I've tried so hard to ride the waves.
mother of Paweł (boy, age 21)	[Motherhood] is the most beautiful thing every mother can have in life, can be confronted with.
mother of Rafał (boy, age 18)	In short, well, I associate work with, with, with . . . my child, well, at least in my case—a deaf child, work, and once again work. Work . . . I mean the kind when you know what's involved—schoolwork, care, development, and so on.
mother of Jurek (boy, age 19)	To be Jurek's mother is to have a life full of surprises.

TABLE 3.   Maternal Metaphors of Hearing Mothers of Deaf Adolescents with
            Very Limited Proficiency in Spoken Polish and Natural Sign Language
            ("No Language") (All Names Changed)

Hearing Mothers of Deaf Adolescents with Very Limited Proficiency in Spoken Polish and Natural Sign Language	Maternal Metaphors: Word, Image, or Sentence (Utterance Quotations)
mother of Ania (girl, age 22)	Like in spring. A short storm, then it passes, passes, and the weather's nice again.
mother of Alina (girl, age 19)	Well, I, too, associate it all the time with sun, flowers, with joy, that's all it [motherhood] reminds me of.
mother of Marian (boy, age 18)	Like a chocolate box full of delicious chocolates. Maybe . . . I've exaggerated, exaggerated, perhaps someone will laugh at me, but they have my permission.
mother of Melania (girl, age 22)	To be Melania's mother is . . . well, I can say that it's a huge, colorful umbrella, so huge that it almost covers . . . also . . . well, with various . . . colors—light, warm and also gray and dark
mother of Ola (girl, age 19)	To be Ola's mother is like being the mother of a normal girl because it's no fairy tale; it's no poetry, either; just like life! Because you can't compare it with any . . . nothing I know of . . .
mother of Kinga (girl, age 18)	Like the sun . . . Like the sun, which is sometimes behind a little cloud, sometimes it showers because that's how it is in life . . . no black vision this, no
mother of Olek (boy, age 19)	I simply feel I'm a child's mother. Well, I don't know, I'm short of words for comparison.
mother of Ela (girl, age 21)	I would compare it [motherhood] to some—I don't know—sort of very hard work, but . . . work . . .
mother of Roma (girl, age 19)	A volcano, sitting on a volcano

Facilitators of the Development of Proficiency in Spoken or Natural Sign Language in Deaf Adolescent Children of Hearing Parents in Light of the Empirical Evidence

In light of the empirical findings presented in this chapter, two theoretically and practically significant determinants of the development of language competence in deaf children of hearing parents can be identified: the mother-child relationship and the mother-father relationship as experienced by mothers.

Analysis of the emotional characteristics of the mother-child relationship revealed that, although deaf adolescents can be very linguistically competent regardless of the language in which they communicate, their mothers have difficulty experiencing their relationship with their offspring within the sphere of deafness, or they may experience this relationship negatively. They also bring into their relationship with their child various emotions and mental states associated with being a mother of a deaf child (metaphors), and these help the children to develop a psychological life of their own. Presumably the deaf children share with their mother emotions and mental states other than those associated with deafness, enabling the child to develop a verbal self (cf. Stern, 1985).

Mothers also share the emotions and experiences they associated with their adolescent children with the children's fathers (as indicated by representations of the mothers' relationship with the children's fathers). Presumably the quality of the mother-father relationship correlates with the development of language competence in deaf adolescents. Mothers share their experiences and emotions relating to the child's deafness with their spouses but not with their children. This shows how lonely deaf adolescents can be in their relationship with their hearing parents. It also helps to explain why deaf adolescents find it so hard to experience themselves as deaf.

Mothers of nonspeaking deaf adolescents who have very limited competence in spoken or natural sign language bring unnamed emotions and mental states into their relationship with their children, ones that are difficult to put into words, or "dead" (metaphors). They thus fail to equip their children psychologically to develop language, a skill that enables the exchange of meaning with other people.

The findings of this study show that we must determine why not every deaf child of hearing parents achieves proficiency in a spoken or natural sign language as a result of the quality of the relationship between the deaf child and the hearing mother.

CONCLUSIONS

The most important clinical implication of the present study is the need to provide mothers of deaf children with various forms of psychological intervention, such as psychoeducation, psychotherapy, and support groups, depending on the type of problems they are experiencing. All mothers need to develop the "motherhood constellation" (Stern, 1995), which is facilitated by the psychotherapeutic relation. This kind of relationship is also essential for mothers of children whose development is more typical (ibid.). This postulate is particularly relevant to hearing mothers of deaf children, and the present findings lend further support to it. The educational and rehabilitative approach, which still dominates in early intervention programs for families with deaf children in many countries, ignores the clinical aspects of the experience of self-as-mother-of-a-deaf-child or may actually support the development of a false maternal identity, self as mother of an "as if hearing" child, "normal" child, or a child "just like other children."

The next postulate is that it would be beneficial to offer parents of deaf children family-oriented interventions in the mother-father-child triad (Jasiński, 2004). According to an educationally oriented perspective (Kushalnagar et al., 2007), such interventions facilitate early communication with the child and initial language development.

Finally, let me quote two comments I heard in Haarlem, where I presented my findings at the annual conference of the European Society for Mental Health and Deafness in 2007. I believe they are important in the context of practical implications. One commentator, a social worker from the South African Republic, suggested the importance of psychological support for the mothers and fathers of deaf children, who need to learn to "talk to each other and share their experiences associated with their child's deafness."

The second comment was made behind the scenes by a hearing mother of three deaf children. She told me that she had "never thought of talking to [her] children about their experiences of deafness because [she] had thought they were so obvious, so normal." It was only when she heard my presentation that she realized "how very important it would be for [her] deaf children to talk about such things with their mother and also how difficult this still was for [her]." These two "voices in the discussion" point to new directions in psychological interventions for hearing parents of deaf children, interventions that could also help deaf children to become proficient in either spoken or natural sign language.

REFERENCES

Allen, T. (1986). Patterns of academic achievement among hearing impaired students. In S. Schildroth & M. Karchmer (Eds.), *Deaf Children in America* (pp. 161–206). San Diego: Little and Brown.

Archbold, S. M. (2005). Paediatric cochlear implantation: Has cochlear implantation changed the face of deaf education? *ENT News, 14*, 52–54.

Barker, P. (1997). *Psychotherapeutic metaphors: Theory and practice* (Polish transl. J. Węgrodzka). Gdańsk: GWP.

Bat-Chava, Y., & Deignan, E. (2001). Peer relationships of children with cochlear implants. *Journal of Deaf Studies and Deaf Education, 6*, 178–189.

Black, P. A., & Glickman, N. S. (2006). Demographics, psychiatric diagnoses, and other characteristics of North American deaf and hard-of-hearing inpatients. *Journal of Deaf Studies and Deaf Education, 11*, 303–321.

Bouvet, D. (1982/1996). *La parole de l'enfant: Pour une éducation bilingue de l'enfant sourd* (Polish transl. R. Gałkowski). Warsaw: WSiP.

Crosson, J., & Geers, A. (2001). Analysis of narrative ability in children with cochlear implants. *Ear & Hearing, 22*, 381–394.

DiFrancesca, S. (1972). *Academic achievement test results of a national testing program for hearing impaired students—United States, Spring* (Series D, No. 9). Washington, DC: Gallaudet College, Office of Demographic Studies.

Fellinger, J., Holzinger, D., Drobner, U., Gerich, J., Lehner, R., Lenz, G., & Goldberg, D. (2005). Mental distress and quality of life in a deaf population. *Social Psychiatry and Psychiatric Epidemiology, 40*, 737–742.

Gacek, M. J. (2007). Kompetencja komunikacyjna niesłyszących gimnazjalistów: Doniesienie z badań [Communication competence in deaf junior high school students: A research report]. *Szkoła Specjalna, 2*, 105–114.

Glickman N. S. (1996). The development of culturally Deaf identities. In N. S. Glickman & M. A. Harvey (Eds.), *Culturally affirmative psychotherapy with Deaf persons* (pp. 115–153). Mahwah, NJ: Erlbaum.

Glickman, N. S. (2007). Do you hear voices? Problems in assessment of mental status in deaf persons with severe language deprivation. *Journal of Deaf Studies and Deaf Education, 12*, 127–147.

Hindley, P. (2000). Child and adolescent psychiatry. In P. Hindley & N. Kitson (Eds.), *Mental health and deafness* (pp. 42–75). London: Whurr.

Janjua, F., Woll, B., & Kyle, J. (2002). Effects of paternal style of interaction on language development in very young severe and profound deaf children. *International Journal of Pediatric Otorhinolaryngology, 64*, 193–205.

Jasiński, T. J. (2004). *Dziecko nie mówi . . . Badanie przymierza rodzinnego w triadzie matka-ojciec-dziecko* [Our child does not speak . . . A study of family collusion in the mother-father-child triad]. Warsaw: Wydawnictwa Uniwersytetu Warszawskiego.

Kamińska, M. (2003). *Wybór sposobu komunikowania się z dzieckiem głuchym mającym słyszących rodziców* [Choosing a mode of communicating with a deaf child of hearing parents]. Unpublished master's thesis, University of Warsaw, Warsaw, Poland.

Kitson, N., & Fry, R. (1990). Prelingual deafness and psychiatry. *British Journal of Hospital Medicine, 44*, 353–356.

Klatter-Folmer, J., Kolen, E., van Hout, R., & Verhoeven, L. (2006). Language development in deaf children's interactions with deaf and hearing adults: A Dutch longitudinal study. *Journal of Deaf Studies and Deaf Education, 11*, 238–251.

Kobosko, J. (2007). *Tożsamość macierzyńska matek słyszących młodzieży głuchej i jej znaczenie dla rozwoju osobowej tożsamości tej młodzieży* [Maternal identity of hearing mothers of deaf adolescents and its significance for the development of young people's personal identity]. Unpublished doctoral dissertation, University of Warsaw, Warsaw, Poland.

Kobosko, J., & Kosmalowa, J. (2000). Depression and the implanted child family. *Fifth European Symposium on Pediatric Cochlear Implantation*, abstract book, Amsterdam.

Kobosko, J., & Zalewska, M. (2011). Maternal identity of hearing mothers of deaf adolescents. Empirical studies: An interpersonal approach. *Volta Review, 111*, 39–59.

Koester, L. S., Brooks, L., & Traci, M. A. (2000). Tactile contact by deaf and hearing mothers during face-to-face interactions with their infants. *Journal of Deaf Studies and Deaf Education, 5*, 127–139.

Koester, L. S., & Meadow-Orlans, K. P. (1991). Parenting a deaf child: Stress, strength and support. In D. F. Moores & K. P. Meadow-Orlans (Eds.), *Educational and developmental aspects of deafness* (pp. 299–320). Washington, DC: Gallaudet University Press.

Krakowiak, K. (2003). Zaburzenia mowy u dzieci z uszkodzeniami słuchu [Speech disorders in children with impaired hearing]. In K. Krakowiak (Ed.), *Szkice o wychowaniu dzieci z uszkodzeniami słuchu* [Essays on the education of children with impaired hearing]. Stalowa Wola, Poland: Wydział Nauk Społecznych KUL.

Kroese, J., Lotz, W., Puffer, C., & Osberger, M. J. (1986). Language and learning skills of hearing impaired children. *ASHA Monographs, 23*, 66–77.

Kushalnagar, P., Mehta, P., Krull, K., Caudle, S., Hannay, J., & Oghalai, J. (2007). Intelligence, parental depression, and behavior adaptability in deaf children being considered for cochlear implantation. *Journal of Deaf Studies and Deaf Education, 12*, 335–349.

Marschark, M., Rothen, C., & Fabich, M. (2007). Effects of cochlear implants on children's reading and academic achievement. *Journal of Deaf Studies and Deaf Education, 12*, 269–282.

Marschark, M., & Spencer, P. E. (Eds.) (2003). *Deaf studies, language, and education* (pp. 151–215). Oxford: Oxford University Press.

Napier, J., & Cornes, A. (2003). The dynamic roles of interpreters and therapists. In S. Austen & S. Crocker (Eds.), *Deafness in mind: Working psychologically with deaf people across the lifespan* (pp. 161–179). London: Whurr.

Novick-Kline, P., Turk, C. L., Mennin, D. S., Hoyt, E. A., & Gallagher, C. L. (2005). Level of emotional awareness as a differentiating variable between individuals with and without generalized anxiety disorder. *Anxiety Disorders, 19*, 557–572.

Pipp-Siegel, S., Sedey, A. L., & Yoshinaga-Itano, C. (2002). Predictors of parental stress in mothers of young children with hearing loss. *Journal of Deaf Studies and Deaf Education, 7*, 1–17.

Preissler, G. (2007). The psychosocial development of deaf children with cochlear implants. In L. Komesaroff (Ed.), *Surgical consent: Bioethics and cochlear implantation* (pp. 120–136). Washington, DC: Gallaudet University Press.

Punch, R., & Hyde, M. B. (2011). Communication, psychosocial and educational outcomes of children with cochlear implants and challenges remaining for professionals and parents. *International Journal of Otolaryngology.* Doi:10.1155/2011/573280

Ricoeur, P. (1990/2005). *Soi-même comme un autre* (Polish transl. B. Chełstowski). Warsaw: Wydawnictwo Naukowe PWN.

Scheetz, N. A. (2004). *Psychosocial aspects of deafness.* Boston: Pearson Education.

Schlesinger, H. S., & Meadow, K. P. (1972). *Sound and sign: Childhood deafness and mental health.* Los Angeles: University of California Press.

Spencer, L. J., Barker, B. A., & Tomblin, J. B. (2003). Exploring the language and literacy outcomes of pediatric cochlear implant users. *Ear & Hearing, 24*, 236–247.

Stern, D. N. (1985). *The interpersonal world of the infant.* New York: Basic Books.

Stern, D. N. (1995). *The motherhood constellation: A unified view of parent-infant psychotherapy.* New York: Basic Books.

Szczygieł, D., & Kolańczyk, A. (2000). Skala Poziomów Świadomości Emocji: Adaptacja skali Levels of Emotional Awareness Scale Lane'a i Schwarza [Polish adaptation of Lane and Schwartz's Levels of Emotional Awareness Scale]. *Roczniki Psychologiczne, 3*, 155–179.

Thoutenhoofd, E. (2006). Cochlear implanted pupils in Scottish schools: 4-year school attainment data (2000–2004). *Journal of Deaf Studies and Deaf Education, 11*, 171–188.

Traxler, C. B. (2000). Measuring up to performance standards in reading and mathematics: Achievement of selected deaf and hard-of-hearing students in the national norming of the 9th Edition Stanford Achievement Test. *Journal of Deaf Studies and Deaf Education, 5*, 337–348.

van Gent, T., Goedhart, A. W., Hindley, P. A., & Treffers, P. D. A. (2007). Prevalence and correlates of psychopathology in a sample of deaf adolescents. *Journal of Child Psychology and Psychiatry, 48*, 950–958.

Wallis, D., Musselman, C., & MacKay, S. (2004). Hearing mothers and their deaf children: The relationship between early, ongoing mode match and subsequent mental health functioning in adolescence. *Journal of Deaf Studies and Deaf Education, 9*, 2–14.

Wojda, P. (2009). Kompetencje w języku migowym u młodzieży głuchej [Natural sign language competence in deaf adolescents]. In J. Kobosko (Ed.), *Młodzież głucha i słabosłysząca w rodzinie i otaczającym świecie: Dla terapeutów, nauczycieli, wychowawców i rodziców* [Deaf and hard of hearing adolescents in the family and the environment: For therapists, teachers, educators, and parents]. Warsaw: Stowarzyszenie "Usłyszeć Świat."

Wojda, P. (2010). Transmission of Polish sign systems. In D. Brentari (Ed.), *Sign languages: A Cambridge Language Survey* (pp. 131–147). Cambridge: Cambridge University Press.

Young, A., & Tattersall, H. (2007). Universal newborn hearing screening and early identification of deafness: Parents' responses to knowing early and their expectations of child communication development. *Journal of Deaf Studies and Deaf Education, 12*, 209–219.

Zalewska, M. (1998a). *Dziecko w autoportrecie z zamalowaną twarzą: Psychiczne mechanizmy zaburzeń rozwoju tożsamości dziecka głuchego i dziecka z opóźnionym rozwojem mowy* [Self-portrait of a child with the face painted over: Psychological mechanisms of identity development disorders of deaf children and children with language delay]. Warsaw: J. Santorski & Wydawnictwo.

Zalewska, M. (1998b). Psychologiczne aspekty stwierdzenia głuchoty u dziecka [Psychological aspects of the diagnosis of deafness in children]. In J. Rola (Ed.), *Wybrane problemy psychologicznej diagnozy zaburzeń rozwoju dzieci* [Selected issues in the psychological diagnosis of developmental disorders in children] (pp. 177–186). Warsaw: Wydawnictwo WSPS.

13

Deafness, Autism, and Diagnostics: A Case Study

Benito Estrada Aranda
Georgina Mitre Fajardo
Ricardo Canal Bedia

For some years, the literature has often addressed autism in deaf people. The diagnosis of autistic spectrum disorders (ASD) is particularly difficult when compounded by the presence of prelocutive, profound deafness, mainly because of the issues surrounding communication problems (Roper, Arnold, & Monteiro, 2003). Until recently, very little was known about deafness and autism in children (Vernon & Rhodes, 2009), but we do know that deaf children with autism present the same symptoms as hearing children with autism, even though the former are usually diagnosed at more advanced ages than the latter (Steinberg, 2008). Autism occurs in approximately 1 out of 80 children with deafness (Gallaudet Research Institute, 2007). A study of autism prevalence in deaf children in the United States during the 2009–2010 school year estimated the incidence of deaf children with autism at 1 out of 53 students (Szymanski, Brice, Lam, & Hotto, 2012). When examining specifically 8-year-old deaf children, the prevalence decreased to 1 out of 59 students (ibid.).

Deaf children with autism and hearing children with autism share the same deficit even though it is provoked by two different causes: a delay or an alteration in oral language development. Absence of a focused intervention in this specific area may contribute to few opportunities to develop their potential, a general sense of isolation, and difficulties with integration into different environments: school, work, family, and so on. They also share the same etiology, such as genetics; maternal exposure to a virus or toxins; complications at birth or during prenatal development; and rubella during pregnancy. However, deaf children who present autism have even more reason to show language delay and difficulties in establishing an efficient communication method (Vernon & Rhodes, 2009).

The simultaneous effects of autism and deafness create a complex life, one that is full of great challenges, especially language development.

To deaf children, the sense of sight (eye contact, joint attention) represents the main access to the world by enabling them to build reality, establish interpersonal relationships, and learn a language. However, when deafness and autism coexist, the sense of sight, although it is not physically affected, can be compromised since pragmatic use is weakened. These children could make eye contact; however, its limited nature can affect the overall quality of the message received or prevent it from being received at all. This singular feature emphasizes the difficulties that could be experienced during the development of persons with multiple disabilities. Deaf children are included in this category because they are at risk of having additional disabilities; in fact, data from the Gallaudet Research Institute indicate that, during the 2009–2010 school year, approximately 40% of deaf children in the United States had additional disabilities (Szymanski, Brice, Lam, & Hotto, 2012).

On the other hand, a child with hearing loss can exhibit behaviors that appear autistic (e.g., not listening or responding when called); social interaction is poor, and isolation and self-stimulation behaviors can develop (Szymanski & Brice, 2008). The deaf child can present with these behaviors, which are also found in autistic disorders, and is thus at risk of being incorrectly diagnosed with autism; as a result, the child may not receive the appropriate attention, treatment, and education.

Regarding the autism-deafness binomial, Gordon (1982, 1999) has proposed the theory that autism could be an unusual variance of peripheral deafness or ear disease even though there is no solid evidence of this. Knoors and Mathijs (2011) explain that other studies have found hearing loss in children with autism. One of these (Klin, 1993) reviewed 11 studies of children and adolescents with autism. Although no clear evidence of brain dysfunction was found, signs of peripheral hearing loss were evident in subjects with autism (ibid.). Percentages of prevalence varied from 13% to 44% (ibid.). Another study (Rosenhall, Nordin, Sandström, Ahlsén, & Gillberg, 1999) identified a 7.9% mild-to-moderate loss of hearing in a group of 199 children and adolescents with autism in Sweden. Profound hearing loss was found in 3.5% of those children, which is significantly higher than in the general population of children, whose percentages of profound hearing loss are typically no higher than 0.1% or 0.2% of all children (Marschark, 1993).

Some authors (e.g., Malandraki & Okalidou, 2007) report that autism can occur more frequently in children as the result of a viral disease that may also affect the ear, such as congenital rubella (Chess, 1971) and congenital cytomegalovirus infection (Stubbs, Ash, & Williams, 1984).

Children who have neither access to communication nor a communication system to represent reality may exhibit deficits in linguistic, communicative, psychological, and social aspects of development due to the isolation this situation creates. In the case of deaf children with autism, these dimensions magnify the diagnostic complexity (Szymanski & Brice, 2008).

Some factors contributing to the difficulty of autism diagnosis in deaf children are delayed language development, social shyness, delays and abnormalities in developing games, interests, and limited activities. While these characteristics are virtually identical to those occurring in hearing children with autism, they could go unnoticed or be incorrectly attributed to characteristics expected of a deaf child (Steinberg, 2008). Studies of autism and deafness (e.g., Roper et al., 2003) have found no difference in the symptomatology of autism in groups of hearing children with autism and groups of deaf children with autism. Nonetheless, the autistic deaf children were diagnosed later than the autistic hearing children (ibid.). The researchers concluded that indicators of autism for both deaf and hearing groups were the same, but in the case of the deaf children, the symptoms were more readily attributed to deafness before being recognized as signs of autism. Additionally, the researchers concluded that the diagnosis of autism in profoundly deaf children is more complex because of shared indicators of developmental delays, such as communication, social abilities, and linguistic skills.

Though, research reveals that autism seems to correlate positively with auditory deficiency (Knoors & Mathijs, 2011; Carvill, 2001). Moreover, because characteristics of autism and deafness are superimposed, some authors (Jure, Rapin, & Tuchman, 1991) have suggested both an underdiagnosis of autism in deaf children and children with auditory deficiencies and an underdiagnosis of auditory deficiencies in children with autism.

At St. Joseph's School for the Deaf in New York, an in-depth study of autism and deafness was conducted with 1,150 deaf students (ibid.). In a sample of 46 students (30 boys and 16 girls), 4 had both autism and deafness. Diagnosis of deafness occurred on average at 2 years of age and of autism at 4 years of age. An interesting result of this study is that the cause of autism in 23 of these 46 students was encephalopathic events: congenital rubella, bacterial meningitis, severe prematurity, and hypoxia, which are also causes of deafness. In six other cases, autism was due to a genetic factor without complications. Vernon and Rhodes (2009) mention studies (Chess, Fernandez, & Korn, 1972; Jure et al., 1991) that have demonstrated that numerous conditions can cause the co-occurrence of autism and deafness: rubella, cytomegalovirus, herpes, chicken pox, toxoplasmosis, syphilis, mumps, prematurity, and hemophiliac influenza. Most of these conditions can cause a significant hearing loss, but they are also likely to cause other disabilities, including some forms of brain damage (Vernon, 1969), contributing to a complex diagnosis.

In another study of deafness and autism, 32,334 deaf and hard of hearing children participated (Szymanski et al., 2012). Data were provided by the 2009–2010 Annual Survey of Deaf and Hard of Hearing Children and Youth, which indicated a total of 37,828 such children registered that year. A total of 12,595 (39.9 %) of all of the deaf children included in the annual survey had an additional disability.

Of this group, 611 children (1.9 %) had a diagnosis of autism in 2009 or 2010. This study reported relevant findings on deafness and autism. For instance, the presence of other relevant conditions, such as developmental delay, intellectual disability, visual weakness, or attention deficit disorders was identified in 58.9% of this sample. Likewise, a high percentage of this sample had a profound hearing loss (> 90 dB), while the remaining sample exhibited lower levels of hearing loss (severe, moderate, etc.), indicating a more severe hearing loss in deaf children with autism than in deaf children without autism (ibid.).significant difference between the severity of hearing loss in deaf children with autism and in deaf children without a diagnosis of autism (ibid.).

DIAGNOSIS

One of the challenges surrounding the diagnosis of autism spectrum disorder (ASD) in deaf children is the availability of an appropriate diagnostic instrument. Some authors indicate that a number of children with autism are psychometrically unstable (Vernon & Rhodes, 2009), an additional factor for the difficulty of having an appropriate diagnostic tool since certain instruments contain items that are inappropriate when applied to deaf children.

Autism diagnosis clearly requires a multidisciplinary evaluation (Le Couteur, Haden, Hammal, & McConachie, 2008). The minimum requirements for an assessment are a valid test for symptomatology associated with autism, a standardized intelligence test, and a standardized adaptive skills test (Palomo, Velayos, Garrido, Tamarit, & Muñoz, 2005). This assessment must also include a detailed history of its development, a description of the child's most frequent behaviors, a cognitive and linguistic evaluation, and detailed observations of how the child is developing in different scenarios (Morris, 2009; cf. Le Couteur et al., 2008; Ozonoff, Goodlin-Jones, & Solomon, 2005). By gathering and integrating information from various sources (e.g., assessment instruments, interviews, observations, registries, opinions from diverse experts), we can work toward reaching a comprehensive differential diagnosis.

Two internationally validated and recognized tests designed for use with symptomatology associated with autism spectrum disorder and autism are the Autism Diagnostic Interview-Revised (ADI-R) (Rutter, Le Couteur, & Lord, 2006) (a parents' interview) and the Autism Diagnostic Observation Schedule (ADOS) (Lord, Rutter, DiLavore, & Risi, 2008) (an observation schedule). Even though the creators of the ADOS do not recommend that test for autism diagnosis in deaf and blind children, it may be used as part of an informal observation. They recommend particularly not using the algorithm since many of the items may be inappropriate; instead, they recommend that a professional opinion be obtained to determine the scope of limitations and their impact on ADOS scoring (ADOS FAQs, 2012).

The following diagnostic instruments can be added to ADI-R and ADOS in order to make a more specific diagnosis when necessary (Morris, 2009):

- Leiter International Performance Scales-Revised (Tsatsanis et al., 2003)
- Mullen Scales of Early Learning (MSEL) (Mullen, 1995)
- Differential Abilities Scales (Elliott, 1990)
- Peabody Picture Vocabulary Test (Dunn & Dunn, 1997)
- Expressive One-Word Picture Vocabulary Test (Brownell, 2000)
- Clinical Evaluation of Language Fundamentals (Semel-Mintz, Wiig, & Secord, 2003)
- Preschool Language Scale (Zimmerman, Steiner, & Pond, 2002)

In cases of deaf children with autism diagnosis, some studies (e.g., Roper et al., 2003) have reported the application of tests such as the Autism Screening Instrument for Educational Planning-2 (ASIEP-2: Krug, Arick, & Almond, 1993), which comprises the Autism Behavior Checklist (ABC) and the Interaction Assessment (IA; Krug, Arick, & Almond, 1980).

Concerning the treatment of deaf children with autism, even though the available intervention methods can help autistic children and deaf children, no research has yet reported a therapy that has been applied to a deaf child with autism (Morris, 2009). Nonetheless, studies (e.g., Malandraki and Okalidou, 2007) have been published on interventions with deaf children with autism utilizing a unique case study design, the Picture Exchange Communication System (PECS) (Morris, 2009). Also available are a study of applied behavioral analysis (Easterbrooks & Handley, 2005) and a study of one family's efforts to help its deaf child with autism (Beals, 2004). Roper et al. (2003) find that the deaf children discussed in these studies were also later diagnosed with autism. Yet another study (Morris, 2009) deals with the relationship between a mother and her deaf child with autism.

The goal of this chapter is to provide data about an informal diagnostic evaluation using the ADI-R and the ADOS carried out on a prelocutive, profoundly deaf child who may be autistic. The purpose is not to determine the diagnosis but to prove that these instruments work with deaf children since, as we have mentioned, the authors do not recommend that ADOS be used on children with profound prelocutive deafness.

METHOD

The design of our research is a unique case study of a prelocutive profoundly deaf child who participated in an in-depth study of prelinguistic skills in deaf children with autism. The teachers at the special education institution where we conducted the study referred to this child as "a deaf child with autism."

SUBJECT

George (pseudonym) is 6 and a half years old and has profound prelocutive deafness. Currently he attends the Center of Multiple Attention, where he receives
special education; he also attends a regular school in the city of Monterrey, Mexico.
George's mother agreed to participate in this study and signed the corresponding
informed-consent form. At present George has behavioral problems: He pesters
other children and used to cry if one of them hit him; he is very playful; he is
always laughing; and he is distracted in class. His mother said that she was worried about George's development, which she had started noticing when he was
3 months old. The first disturbing symptom was that George's head moved backward; when he was 7 months old, his parents called to him, but he did not turn
toward them; he did not crawl, walk, or stand up; he was very quiet, and he did
not cry. Around 2 years of age, George did not play, and he did not communicate. Learning to walk was difficult for him; finally he started walking normally
and continued doing so until he was 5 years old; now he walks sideways, and
his head still moves backward. At 3 years of age, he was not capable of communicating; he did not play; he ate a lot and did not show any interest in other
children. He was toilet trained at 3 years of age, and at 4 years he had no toilet-
training accidents for 12 months. Also at 4 years of age he said his first words:
"daddy," "peanut," "breath." He confused "daddy" and "mom." At 6 years of
age he started forming phrases by joining simple words (e.g., "I want water,"
"eat egg," "eat cheese"). George's mother states that he did generally did not
look at her but that sometimes he gazes absently at her; similarly, it is hard to get
his attention. His mother reports that when George entered elementary school,
his behavior grew worse. He understands few words if his mother does not use
signs or gestures.

George's mother recognizes that her son does not have a functional use of language since he has no spontaneous phrases of more than three words. Regarding
his sign language, she reports that she does not understand him when he makes
signs, and he used to confuse "I" and "you." He teaches sign language to his little dog. When George wants something, he points to it to indicate that someone
should bring it to him; however, he does not look at the person, and he does not
combine gestures with sounds. Sometimes George holds the other person's wrist
to indicate something he is interested in. He makes some facial expressions when
he is having fun; for example, he is capable of smiling; however, his mother told us
she feels he is not able to show a variety of expressions as do other children of his
age. Sometimes he makes facial expressions that are inappropriate for a particular
situation, and up to 4–5 years of age, George did not play with his toys but en-
joyed messing them up repeatedly. He generally does not play with other children
but prefers to play by himself. In earlier stages, George formed an attachment to

various objects: shoes, a pair of socks, a toy house he did not play with; he also had a special interest in playing with tires, rocks, and tamarind balls and in lining cards up according to colors. He likes to pick up objects of the same category. Sometimes he is especially interested in smelling things and people.

PROCEDURE

Once informed written consent was obtained from the subject's mother, as well as authorization from the institution he was attending, psychometric testing started. In some sessions, assessments were carried out in a cubicle at the institution during school hours. The cubicle was equipped with furniture that allowed us to work with George. Similarly, it had good lighting and limited visual stimuli, which allowed greater participant concentration. Of their own volition, neither the mother nor the institution personnel were present during George's sessions, believing this configuration to be more beneficial to George.

During the first session, we administered the Merrill-Palmer-Revised Scales of Development, which assess cognition, fine motor skills, and receptive language and include supplementary scales that evaluate memory, speed, and visuomotor skills. These scales, which lasted approximately 60 minutes, were administered by a specialized examiner in Mexican Sign Language. During the second session, George was administered the 50-minute ADOS. Because of its length, the ADI-R interview was conducted in two sessions with the mother present. The mother's interview was carried out in another part of the institution. Two examiners participated in these assessments.

Instruments

The Merrill-Palmer-R Scales of Development
(Roid & Sampers, 2004)

This scale was designed for early identification of developmental delay and learning problems in children from 1 to 78 months of age. These assessments are required by state and federal legislation in the United States. This scale may also be utilized to evaluate children with regard to auditory deficiency, autism, or other cases of limited expressive language. As mentioned earlier, this scale measures cognitive development, fine motor skills, and receptive language and provides several other supplementary tests. The administration of this scale takes 30 to 40 minutes. The scale was standardized by a national representative sample of 1,068 children selected by gender, ethnic group, parents' educational level, and geographical region per the 2000 census (U.S. Bureau of the Census, 2001).

Autism Diagnostic Interview-Revised (ADI-R; Rutter et al., 2006)

The ADI-R consists of a semistructured interview administered to parents. The interview elicits information from the parents about their child's behavior. It comprises 93 questions and takes 2 to 3 hours to administer. The ADI-R covers primarily three domains—language and communication, social interactions and behavior, and restricted, repetitive, or stereotyped interests—which are the three functional domains that have been identified as important diagnostic elements both in the International Classification of Diseases (ICD) (WHO, 1992) and in the DSM-5 (American Psychiatric Association, 2013). The evaluated subject (absent during the interview) must have attained the development characteristic of at least a 2-year- and 0-month-old child regardless of the subject's conditions and chronological age. Among the population groups for whom the ADI-R is appropriate are children with severe developmental language disorders, especially those involving receptive difficulties (Howlin, Mawhood, & Rutter, 2000). During the interview we made adjustments to some of the questions, mainly in the categories of "acquisition and loss of language/other skills" and "working with the language and communication," according to the particular characteristics of George's language, which consisted primarily of signs.

Autism Diagnostic Observation Schedule

The Autism Diagnostic Observation Schedule (ADOS; Lord et al., 2008) is a semistructured, standardized test of communication, social interaction, and play or material imaginative use. It obtains information by directly observing individual behaviors in a variety of activities and elicited behaviors. This scale comprises four different modules, one of which must be selected so as to be applied according to the level of expressive language of the subject, and typically takes 30 to 45 minutes to administer. Modules 1 and 2 are administered while constant movement is occurring in the room, according to interests and activities appropriate for young children or those with very limited language ability; modules 3 and 4 are carried out sitting at a table, implying more conversation and language without a specific physical context (ibid.). This scale may be applied to persons who have a mental age of more than 2 years. During our administration of the ADOS, modifications were made in the presentation of the established models in order to accommodate deafness. For example, item 2 ("Answer by name") was adapted by saying "George" and touching George's shoulder; this had mixed success. Item 3 ("Responding to joint attention") attempts to get a child's attention by making a hand movement, similar to the way that people will say someone's name to get the person's attention. After getting George's attention, we began the process of looking at an object (toy) in an attempt to elicit joint attention.

RESULTS

The Merrill-Palmer-Revised (MPR) cognitive battery was designed to measure a multifaceted model of cognitive skills, fine motor skills, and receptive language (Roid & Sampers, 2004). The combination of the scores of these individual skills generates an overall score, which is called the development index (DI) (see Table 1). George presents a DI equivalent to that of a 33-month-old child, as well as a cognitive index equivalent to that of a 38-month-old child. He exhibits a serious delay in development according to a descriptive classification of DI levels and domain scores per the MPR. We observed that George has a low level of receptive language compared to the other domains included in the DI; therefore, we believe his deafness conditions may be significantly and negatively influencing his global development.

According to the results obtained from the ADI-R, whose purpose is to obtain sufficient information to make (or rule out) a diagnosis of autism, we identified qualitative alteration of social interaction and alterations in development that are evident at 36 months or earlier; we obtained scores higher than the cutoff points established to make a diagnosis of autism (see Table 2). However, a component of the qualitative alteration of communication obtained a score in the limit, and the restricted, repetitive, and stereotyped behavior patterns component was below the cutoff point.

ADOS was also applied to George. During the administration of module 1 we noticed that George was capable of performing the activities appropriately.

The observational scale for autism diagnosis comprises 5 main areas to be assessed, and each one of them is divided into different preverbal skills that indicate

TABLE 1. Merrill Palmer Scales of Development-Revised (Cognitive Battery)

Domains	Raw Score	Growth Score	Age Equivalent (in months)	Percentiles	Standard Score
developmental index	166	437	33	< 0.1	25
cognitive	75	443	38	0.1	51
fine motor skills	49	455	50	0.3	58
receptive language	41	420	30	< 0.1	16
Supplemental Scores					
memory	13	440	36	< 0.1	40
speed	15	467	58	4.8	75
visuomotor skills	45	451	44	< 0.1	43

TABLE 2.   Scores Obtained in Domains: ADI-R Diagnostic Algorithm

Domains		Scores	Cutoff Points
Domain A. reciprocal social interaction qualitative alterations		13	10
Domain B. communication qualitative alterations	total verbal B (V)		8
	total verbal B (NV)	7	7
Domain C. restricted repeated and stereotyped behavioral patterns		2	3
Domain D. evident developmental alterations up to 36 months		3	1

Note. V = verbal; NV = nonverbal

TABLE 3.   Scores Obtained in Domains: ADOS Diagnostic Algorithm

Domains	Scores	Cutoff Points	
	autism	autistic	spectrum
A. communication	4	4	2
B. reciprocal social interaction	3	7	4
total of communication + reciprocal social interaction	7	12	
C. play		7	
D. stereotyped and restricted interests	0		

the presence or absence of recurrent behaviors that fall within the autistic spectrum (see Table 3). This information will help us formulate a diagnosis.

The 5 main areas to be assessed are as follows:

1. Language and communication
2. Reciprocal social interaction
3. Play
4. Stereotyped behaviors and restricted interests
5. Other abnormal behaviors

George clearly engages in symbolic and functional play with appropriate objects, and he is creative when playing; he also functions communicatively through sign language. He is capable of asking for an object or for help in obtaining something; he is capable of sharing emotions and interests; and he succeeded at functional and symbolic imitation. Similarly, George shows interest in a variety of objects, but he also shifts his attention from one object to another without showing unusual interest in any of them; however, he showed no interest in the components of objects.

George obtained scores of 4 in communication and 3 in reciprocal social interaction; in play, 0; and in stereotyped behaviors and restricted interests, 0. The sum of the "communication" and "reciprocal social interaction" scores was thus 7, which is before the cutoff point for autistic spectrum but not for autism as such. However, because of a caveat from the creators of the ADOS regarding its use with deaf or blind persons, we wanted to analyze George's results in detail and adapt them to this particular case. As mentioned earlier, Lord et al. (2008) recommend that the diagnostic algorithm of the ADOS not be used with this cohort because many of the items may not be appropriate; they recommend instead that a professional opinion be obtained to determine the scope of limitations and their impact on ADOS scores (ADOS FAQs, 2012).

CONCLUSIONS

As we have seen, diagnosis of autism for a prelocutive profoundly deaf child may present a challenge due to the coexistence of etiology of both conditions; as such, the symptomatology of one condition may disguise that of the other. As we saw, independent play, shyness, or social isolation, delay in verbal language development, as well as restricted activities and interests are only some of the most frequent and similar symptoms of both conditions. In addition, most diagnostic instruments for autism have been designed for hearing children, which implies a considerable degree of complication in the case of deaf children due to the common difficulties in language development. At presently we do not have instruments designed specifically for diagnosing autism in prelocutive profoundly deaf children (Szymanski & Brice, 2008), which highlights an important psychodiagnostic need.

In the case of the child we studied, although the diagnostic evaluation was carried out using two of the most prestigious and widely used tools to diagnose autism in hearing children, it is difficult to be certain that we have made a sound diagnosis inasmuch as deafness and autism have many observable similarities.

During ADI-R administration, we obtained mixed results; that is, several criteria were achieved, but others were not. Mixed results may have different interpretations. Some researchers have agreed to make an autism diagnosis if scores are clearly above cutoff point in at least two of three domains (A, B, and C behavior domains) and if the difference does not exceed one point in the third domain; others prefer to rule out a diagnosis of autism in cases in which all of the criteria are accomplished (Rutter, LeCouteur, & Lord, 2006). However, the information from direct observations during administration of the ADOS is necessary to confirm possible conclusions when obtaining mixed results. Based on the two options suggested by the researchers for mixed results, we obtained a negative autism diagnosis using the ADI-R. Only one of the A, B, and C behavior domains is clearly above the cutoff specified for autism diagnosis: qualitative alterations of reciprocal social interaction.

On the other hand, when interpreting ADOS results, it is important to understand the meaning of cutoff points (Lord et al., 2008). An individual may obtain a score that falls within the scoring range for a high proportion of individuals with autism and similar types of expressive language disorders. These similarities appear when considering speech and gestures as components of social interaction (communication domain) and of social reciprocity (reciprocal social interaction domain) (ibid.). However, in order to comply completely with the formal criteria for a diagnosis of autism, the subject must also show restricted, repetitive behaviors and meet the onset-age criteria.

Unlike other measures based on information provided by the parents, such as ADI-R or CARS (Schopler, Reichler, De Vellis, & Daly, 1980), ADOS provides a measure only of current performance. Thus, the presence of some behavior in the past (in George's case, the presence of behaviors such as the repetitive use of objects or his interest in the components of objects) may not be considered or constitute part of the scores resulting from the ADOS. They will therefore not cause confusion when integrating the general results. For these reasons, Schopler et al. (ibid.) decided that in order to make a diagnosis of autism spectrum disorder based on the results of the ADOS, subjects must obtain scores equal to or higher than the cutoff points both in the "reciprocal social interaction" domain and the "communication" domain. Under these criteria, we conclude that the data obtained on the past and current performance of George not allow us to say that this child meets all the criteria for a diagnosis of ASD at the time of the assessment. This is despite his having obtained scores higher than the cutoff in the communication domain and in "total of communication + reciprocal social interaction."

We believe that George's score in the domain of communication, which places him in the autistic spectrum, is directly affected by his hearing condition (deafness), remembering as well that Lord et al. (2008) affirm cutoff points that were established according to a high proportion of autistic subjects with similar levels of expressive language difficulties, a condition not present in George's case since his main method of communication is sign language. Frequency of "vocalizations" (signs) addressed to others, pointing out of objects of interest, and gestures were three criteria to be evaluated, and these results placed George in the autistic spectrum. However, these characteristics may differ importantly between deaf and hearing persons; therefore, we acknowledge the possibility that, according this evaluation scale, these characteristics may inadvertently place George in the wrong category.

Likewise, ADOS considers it important to recognize a subject who cannot reconcile ADOS criteria for both autism and ASD even though accentuated abnormalities were present in other areas. Such is the case with George, who obtained outstanding scores in the communication domain. The ADOS suggests that high scores in the reciprocal social interaction or communication domains indicate clinically significant difficulties that will require more study and attention even if they do not reach the cutoff point for diagnostic classification (Lord et al., 2008).

In summary, we believe that, according to the ADOS and the ADI-R results, George has not autism; his scores do not fall in the autistic spectrum, nor do they meet DSM-IV and DSM-5 diagnostic criteria for autistic disorder (this study was conducted before the publication of when DSM-5). A DSM-IV (American Psychological Association, 1996) diagnosis is based on the following categories:

1. Qualitative alteration of social interaction
2. Qualitative alteration of communication
3. Behavior patterns, interests, and restricted, repetitive, and stereotyped activities

Diagnosis is also based on delay or abnormal performance in at least one of the following areas, with onset prior to age 3 years: social interaction; language used in social communication; and symbolic or imaginative play. Moreover, the disorder is not better explained in the presence of Rett syndrome or of infantile disintegrative disorder.

Based on the results and as discussed, we believe that George may not have received the appropriate education and/or pertinent social or educational treatment. Moreover, we believe that deafness enables the appearance of behaviors characteristic of autism, which ends when implementing alternative communication systems (Polaino-Lorente, 1982). George must receive more linguistic stimulation in both sign language and a spoken language.

REFERENCES

ADOS FAQs. (2012). *General Questions: Training, Reliability, Becoming a Trainer, Translation. Can the ADOS be used with children consulted?* Retrieved February 6, 2012, from http://portal .wpspublish.com/portal/page?_pageid=53,84992&_da d=portal&_schema=PORTAL#

American Psychiatric Association. (1996). *Diagnostic and statistical manual of mental disorders* (DSM-IV). Washington, DC: Author.

American Psychiatric Association. (2013). *Diagnostic and statistical manual of mental disorders* (DSM-5). Washington, DC: Author.

Baron-Cohen, S., Allen, J., & Gillberg, C. (1992). Can autism be detected at 18 months? The needle, the haystack and the CHAT. *British Journal of Psychiatry, 161,* 839–843.

Beals, K. (2004). Early intervention in deafness and autism: One family's experiences, reflections, and recommendations. *Infants and Young Children, 17,* 284–290.

Brownell, R. (2000). *Expressive one-word picture vocabulary test* (3rd ed.). Novato, CA: Academic Therapy Publications.

Carvill, S. (2001). Sensory impairments, intellectual disability and psychiatric. *Journal of Intellectual Disability Research, 45*(6), 467–483.

Chess, S. (1971). Autism in children with congenital rubella. *Journal of Autism and Childhood Schizophrenia, 1*, 33–47.

Chess, S., Fernandez, P., & Korn, S. J. (1972). *Psychiatric disorders in children with congenital rubella.* New York: Brunner Mazel.

Dunn, L. M., & Dunn, L. M. (1997). *Peabody Picture Vocabulary Test* (3rd ed.). Circle Pines, MN: American Guidance Service.

Easterbrooks, S. R., & Handley, C. M. (2005). Behavior change in a student with a dual diagnosis of deafness and pervasive developmental disorder: A case study. *American Annals of the Deaf, 150,* 401–407.

Elliott, C. D. (1990). *Differential abilities scales: Administration and scoring manual.* San Antonio, TX: Psychological Press.

Gallaudet Research Institute. (2007). *Regional and national summary report of data from the 2006–2007 Annual Survey of Deaf and Hard of Hearing Children and Youth.* Washington, DC: Author.

Gordon, A. G. (1982). Does anyone read old medical journals? (Letter). *American Journal of Psychiatry, 139*(2), 259-a-259. http://dx.doi.org/10.1176/ajp.139.2.259-a

Gordon, A. G. (1999). Understanding autism: Does anyone read new medical journals? *Journal of Psychiatry & Neuroscience, 24*(4), 352.

Howlin, P., Mawhood, L., & Rutter, M. (2000). Autism and developmental receptive language disorder—a follow-up comparison in early adult life. II: Social, behavioural, and psychiatric outcomes. *Journal of Child Psychology and Psychiatry, and Allied Disciplines, 41*(5), 561–578.

Jure, R., Rapin, I., & Tuchman, R. (1991). Hearing impaired autistic children. *Developmental Medicine and Child Neurology, 33*(12), 1062–1072.

Klin, A. (1993). Auditory brainstem responses in autism: Brainstem dysfunction or peripheral hearing loss? *Journal of Autism and Developmental Disorders, 23*(1), 15–35.

Knoors, H., & Mathijs, P. J. (2011). Educational programming for deaf children with multiple disabilities: Accommodating special needs. In M. Marschark and P. E. Spencer (Eds.), *Oxford Handbook of Deaf Studies, Language, and Education, Vol. 1* (2nd ed.) 82–96. doi: 10.1093/oxfordhb/9780199750986.013.0007

Krug, D. A., Arick, J. R., & Almond, P. J. (1980). Behaviour checklist for identifying severely handicapped individuals with high levels of autistic behaviour. *Journal of Child Psychology and Psychiatry, 21,* 221–229.

Krug, D. A., Arick, J. R., & Almond, P. J. (1993). *Autism screening instrument for educational planning* (2nd ed.). Examiner's manual. Portland, OR: ASIEP Education.

Le Couteur, H. G., Haden, G., Hammal, D., & McConachie, H. (2008). Diagnosing autism spectrum disorders in pre-school children using two standardised assessment instruments: The ADI-R and the ADOS. *Journal of Autism and Developmental Disorders, 38,* 362–372.

Lord, C., Rutter, M., DiLavore, P. C., & Risi, S. (2008). *Escala de observación para el diagnóstico del autismo* [Autism Diagnostic Observation Schedule]. Madrid: TEA Ediciones.

Malandraki, G., & Okalidou, A. (2007). The application of PECS in a deaf child with autism: A case study. *Focus on Autism and Other Development Disability, 22,* 23. doi: 10.1177/10883576070220010301

Marschark, M. (1993). *Psychological development of deaf children.* New York: Oxford University Press.

Morris, P. A. (2009). *My deaf autistic son and me.* Master's thesis, Queen's University, Ontario, Canada.

Mullen, E. (1995). Mullen Scales of Early Learning. Circle Pines, MN: American Guidance Service.

Ozonoff, S., Goodlin-Jones, B. L., & Solomon, M. (2005). Evidence-based assessment of autism spectrum disorders in children and adolescents. *Journal of Clinical Child and Adolescent Psychology, 34,* 523–540.

Palomo, R., Velayos, L., Garrido, M. J., Tamarit, J., & Muñoz, A. (2005). Evaluación y diagnóstico en trastornos del espectro de autismo: El modelo IRIDIA. In D. Valdez (Ed.), *Evaluar e intervenir en autismo.* Madrid: Machado Libros.

Polaino-Lorente, A. (1982). *Introducción al estudio científico del autismo infantil.* Madrid: Alambra.

Roid, G. H., & Sampers, J. L. (2004). Merrill-Palmer-R: Scales of Development. Wood Dale, IL: Stoelting.

Roper, L., Arnold, P., & Monteiro, B. (2003). Co-occurrence of autism and deafness. *Autism, 7*(3), 245–253.

Rosenhall, U., Nordin, V., Sandstrom, M., Ahlsen, G., & Gillberg, C. (1999). Autism and hearing loss. *Journal of Autism Developmental Disorders, 29*(5), 349–357.

Rutter, M., LeCouteur, A., & Lord, C. (2006). *Entrevista para el diagnóstico del autismo* (Rev. ed.). Madrid: TEA Ediciones.

Schopler, E., Reichler, R., De Vellis, R., & Daly, K. (1980). Toward objective classification of childhood autism: Childhood Autism Rating Scale (CARS). *Journal of Autism and Developmental Disorders, 10,* 91–103.

Semel-Mintz, E., Wiig, E., & Secord, W. (2003). Clinical evaluation of language fundamentals (4th ed.). San Antonio, TX: Psychological Corporation.

Steinberg, G. A. (2008). Understanding the need for language: An introduction to the *Odyssey* special issue on autism and deafness. *Odyssey, 9*(1), 6–9.

Stubbs, G. E., Ash, E., & Williams, C. P. S. (1984). Autism and congenital cytomegalovirus. *Journal of Autism and developmental Disorders, 14,* 183–189.

Szymanski, A. C., & Brice, J. P. (2008). When autism and deafness coexist in children: What we know now. *Odyssey: New Directions in Deaf Education, 9*(1), 10–15.

Szymanski, A. C., Brice, J. P., Lam, H. K., & Hotto, A. S. (2012). Deaf children with autism spectrum disorders. *Journal of Autism Development Disorder, 42*(10), 2027–2037. doi 10.1007/s10803-012-1452-9

Tsatsanis, K. D., Dartnall, N., Cicchetti, D., Sparrow, S. S., Klin, A., & Volkmar, F. R. (2003). Concurrent validity and classification accuracy of the Leiter and Leiter-R in low-functioning children with autism. *Journal of Autism and Developmental Disorders, 33,* 23–30.

U.S. Bureau of the Census. (2001). *Appendix A: Census 2000 geographic terms and concepts.* Retrieved April 5, 2004, from https://www.census.gov/housing/patterns/about/glossary2.pdf

Vernon, M. (1969). Multiple-handicapped deaf children: Medical education and psychological considerations. Reston, VA: Council for Exceptional Children.

Vernon, M., & Rhodes, A. (2009). Deafness and autistic spectrum disorders. *American Annals of the Deaf, 154*(1), 5–14.

World Health Organization (WHO). (1992). The ICD-10 classification of mental and behavioural disorders: Clinical descriptions and diagnostic guidelines. Geneva: Author.

Zimmerman, I. L., Steiner, V. G., & Pond, R. E. (2002). *Preschool Language Scale* (4th ed.). San Antonio, TX: Psychological Corporation.

Final Conclusions

Mental health and deafness is not just a specialization within the field. It is rapidly becoming acknowledged as a complex issue that involves people who are members of minority groups and are at constant risk of social exclusion and having their human rights violated. In the past 30 years, countries such as Holland, England, France, Belgium, Switzerland, Spain, and the United States have developed public mental health services that have been designed to better meet the needs of deaf people. However, these services are not available in most other countries, including Mexico, the home of the Fifth World Congress on Mental Health and Deafness. It is unfortunate that the host country of this international forum does not yet have a specialized, accessible network of public mental health services for its deaf residents.

This book presents a compilation of international research by members and friends of the worldwide Deaf community for the benefit of that community. The right to health is a human right recognized and protected by international rules that nations are obligated to uphold, thus respecting and protecting the right to health of their citizens, who include deaf persons and other minority groups.

We draw attention to the fact that, globally, these rights may not be recognized for persons with disabilities. Many developed countries have laws that protect the human rights of these people, and public and private institutions work to ensure the implementation of these laws. Nonetheless, in other countries these human rights may exist only on the paper on which they were written. Access to health care in a trustful relationship free of communication barriers and respectful of Deaf culture can be regarded as a basic right of Deaf people and the foundation of the necessary respect for human rights. Much work remains to be done, and the human rights chapter in this book is one effort in the continuing insistence on the need for individual countries to make a social and political commitment to ensure due respect for and observance of the basic human rights of deaf people and others with disabilities.

These rights to health for Deaf people must protect them from suffering direct or indirect discrimination as they seek professional health care. But the Deaf community cannot do this alone; it needs the support of the legal framework and the public health policies of their country, which must understand that proper health care for Deaf people with mental disorders is an ethical issue and a human rights question, not a matter of cost-effectiveness.

The topic of human rights is relevant to the lack of mental health services for deaf people in Mexico, a country where such services have not existed until recently. The paucity of demographic and epidemiological information about the Deaf population there, its inadequate access to education and other public services, and the dearth of employment opportunities all constitute severe human rights violations. Unfortunately, this reality is still the status quo in most countries.

We know that, historically, Deaf people have been marginalized and treated as pariahs, but, like hearing people, they can become mentally ill and in some cases require psychiatric treatment. This means that mental health professionals need to be trained and skilled in various aspects of the deaf person's experience: communication and language choices and their impact, medical and developmental complexities and influences, and social, cultural, and emotional issues. Familiarity with these factors is vital to the accurate diagnosis and treatment of Deaf persons. Deaf staff are also a critical element in providing services that are culturally accessible and inviting to potential patients.

With respect to the pharmaceutical treatment of mental illness within the deaf and hard of hearing population, specific psychopharmacological research on this clientele is severely lacking. For this reason, psychiatrists need to be aware of these patients' potentially greater sensitivity to medication, including undesired and often serious side effects. A thorough knowledge of the application, effects, side effects, contraindications, and interactions with other medications is utterly essential.

Regarding cochlear implants and the mental health of deaf recipients, medical researchers have long desired to develop ways to remedy hearing loss, seeing this as a means of integrating deaf and hard of hearing individuals into the mainstream of society. As Irene Leigh states in her chapter, it is time to end the either-or paradigm: either cochlear implantee or culturally Deaf.[1] Within this paradigm, parents' perceptions and general conclusions indicate that they perceive their children as experiencing an improved quality of life, greater self-esteem, more confidence, and more outgoing behavior compared to preimplant. Also, Leigh presents the perspectives of pediatric cochlear implant users. We saw that children with cochlear implants observed in group situations or classroom discourse with hearing peers encounter comparatively more challenges than their hearing peers in their attempts to become active group participants. So, as we see, the cochlear implant does not change the reality of the deaf child immediately; numerous other aspects must also be considered. As Irene concluded, many of the participants with cochlear implants in the studies mentioned earlier rely on spoken language,

thus raising questions about how they label themselves in the deaf-hearing identity domain. It is intriguing that a piece of technology could have the power to
influence one's identity—the sense of who one is.

We also learned of some new treatment that may prove helpful to Deaf people
who need mental health treatment (e.g., eye movement desensitization and reprocessing [EMDR] therapy).[2] In such treatment, EMDR can be effective, given its
compatibility with deaf individuals' distinctive ways of storing and processing
critical events such as communication and social interpretation skills, as well as
family relationship problems. As this book explains, these matters can be quickly
addressed in therapy with deaf clients with the effective contribution of EMDR.

Another unique treatment modality is equine assisted counseling (EAC),
which this book illustrates as a viable and an effective mode of treatment for use
with Deaf individuals, groups, and families. With some modifications to accommodate language, visual accessibility, and cultural sensitivity, this growing field can
offer unique opportunities to a minority group that is often overlooked or swept
aside in the face of clinical innovations and advances. As with hearing clients, Deaf
EAC clients have an opportunity to improve their social-emotional functioning
and gain beneficial insights. It is anticipated that Deaf clients and their families
would continue to benefit from this evolving approach, and future research hopes
to substantiate that.

The correlation between self-esteem and cultural identity was examined, as
well as possible relationships among self-esteem, cultural identity, and selected
demographic factors (age of onset, schooling, communication mode) in deaf and
hard of hearing adults in Cyprus and Greece. The study showed that these adults
generally displayed positive self-esteem and tended to prefer a bicultural identity.
We also confirmed that individuals who were born deaf tended to identify better
with the Deaf community, in contrast to those who reported receiving instruction
in general educational settings or communicating orally with their parents and
other family members, who tended to identify more with the hearing community.
Parents are instrumental in determining their child's identity development, and
exposing one's Deaf children to a well-rounded bicultural environment appears to
facilitate their growth into well-adjusted adults.

Another chapter discussed the quality of life of marginalized minorities such
as the Latino deaf and hard of hearing individuals in the United States. The
chapter points to the importance of parental involvement, family communication, cultural background, and socioeconomic status, all of which influence the
way in which Latino deaf and hard of hearing youth view both their parents'
contribution to their quality of life and their interaction with peers who are
similar to or different from them. An understanding of how these Latino youth
perceive the impact of familial language differences on their quality of life is
important to psychologists, health-care providers, and school personnel, who
will be able to work more effectively with these young people and their parents

to foster and maintain a positive quality of life in general. This chapter explains how language access, parental involvement, and quality family communication can not only influence the development of positive self-esteem and a satisfying quality of life but also foster respect for family heritage, customs, and experiences in another country.

Other subjects discussed in the book are epidemiology, etiology, and cultural, linguistic, and developmental issues, as well as psychopathology as it relates to the Deaf population. Although these topics have been studied for several decades, they continue to perpetuate a number of prejudices and prompt overestimations of the prevalence of certain mental disorders in this group. Thus further epidemiological investigations to gather more accurate data are still needed. Another as yet unsolved problem is the complete absence of specialized psychological and psychiatric assessment services for deaf patients in many countries. Because of this, epidemiological reports on the mental health problems of deaf people around the world continue to be skewed.

The chapter that treats this topic also concludes that it is necessary to offer parents of deaf children family-oriented interventions in the mother-father-child triad because, "according to an educationally oriented perspective," such interventions facilitate early communication with the child and initial language development. This conclusion situates communication as the primary focus of deaf children's development and underlines the decisive role of hearing parents in this process. The chapter also emphasizes the importance of sign language and other forms of communication relevant to the specific needs and resources of each deaf child. In addition, it may also be necessary to provide psychological support for the hearing parents of deaf children because of the typical lack of access to appropriate communication.

Finally, with regard to the overlap between deafness and other disabilities, we still know very little about autism in deaf children. The principal problem with deaf children and autistic children is the coexistence of both conditions. This is the main cause of misdiagnosis since the symptomatology of one condition may disguise the other. As we have seen, independent play, shyness, social isolation, delay in verbal language development, and restricted activities and interests are only some of the most frequent symptoms of both conditions. Moreover, most of the diagnostic instruments for autism have been designed for use with hearing children, which implies a considerable degree of complication in the case of Deaf children due to their different language development. Up to now, we have not had instruments designed specifically for diagnosing autism in prelocutive profoundly deaf children,[3] which highlights an important psychodiagnostic need. Given this situation, in these cases it is difficult to be certain that we have made an accurate diagnosis.

NOTES

1. M. Hintermair & J. Albertini (2005), Ethics, deafness, and new medical technologies. *Journal of Deaf Studies and Deaf Education, 10*(2), 185–192.

2. F. Shapiro (2001), *Eye movement desensitization and reprocessing: Basic principles, protocols and procedures.* New York: Guilford Press.

3. A. C. Szymanski & J. P. Brice (2008), When autism and deafness coexist in children: What we know now. *Odyssey: New Directions in Deaf Education, 9*(1), 10–15.

Contributors

KATERINA ANTONOPOULOU, PH.D, is an assistant professor in learning and communication in the Department of Home Economics and Ecology of Harokopio University in Greece. She has teaching experience in the education of children and adolescents with special educational needs. She has recently published papers on parenting and sibling relationships in families with deaf and hard of hearing children. She is also interested in the study of the development of referential communication and social understanding in deaf and hard of hearing populations.

RICARDO C. BEDIA, PH.D., is a professor in the Department of Personality, Assessment and Psychological Treatment, Instituto Universitario de Integración en la Comunidad (INICO), Universidad de Salamanca (Spain).

MARIA CHARALAMBOUS is a Cyprus Sign Language (CSL) Interpreter, and a M.Ed. holder in special (inclusive) education.

LIEKE DOORNKATE is a psychotherapist, EMDR practioner, and CBT-therapist. Since 1994 she has worked in outpatient mental health and is specialized in the treatment of deaf and hard of hearing clients and their family members. As she is fluent in Dutch Sign Language, treatment is provided to clients in their own language. Since 2010 she has treated deaf and hearing clients in private practice in Amsterdam. In an inspiring cooperation with Jeantine Janse, a Deaf CBT-therapist, she trains new professionals in the field of mental health and deafness.

MELISSA DRAGANAC-HAWK is a first-generation American of Deaf immigrant Peruvian parents. She is the principal of early childhood education at the Pennsylvania School for the Deaf and an adjunct professor of American Sign Language at the University of Pennsylvania. She is a past president of the National Council of Hispano Deaf and Hard of Hearing, and a consultant to the Tri-State Latino Deaf Association.

BENITO ESTRADA ARANDA, PH.D., has a Ph.D. and master's degree in systemic therapy from the Pontifical University of Salamanca (Spain) and a degree in psychology from the Universidad Autonoma de San Luis Potosi (Mexico). He is a full-time research professor at the Psychology School of the University Autonoma of San Luis Potosi. He is a member of the National System of Researchers (Systema Nacional de Investigadores) and has published numerous scientific articles in peer-reviewed international and national journals. He is also the author of several books and book chapters. He is currently involved in funded research and collaborative projects with academic leaders in Mexico and around the world. He was the president of the fifth World Congress on Mental Health and Deafness.

JOHANNES FELLINGER, M.D., PH.D., is head of the Health Centre for the Deaf, Institute of Neurology of Senses and Language at the Hospital of St. John of God, Linz, Austria. He is also a consultant for neurology and psychiatry, neuropediatrics, and an assistant professor for psychiatry 2011 at the University of Vienna. He served the World Federation of the Deaf Expert on Mental Health 2009–2011, and coordinates health issues since 2013. He initiated health and mental health services for the Deaf in Austria (Linz 1991, Vienna 1999, Salzburg 1999, Graz 2007) Bratislava 2008 Lebenswelt Schenkenfelden (a unit for deaf people with multiple disabilities) 1999, a training program for deaf care workers in 1997, and early intervention programs for deaf children. Dr. Fellinger was president of the fifth European Society for Mental Health and Deafness (ESMHD) Congress in 2003, chair of the special interest group, "Public Health" of ESMHD and member of the executive committee. He is a lecturer at the Medical University Vienna, and has conducted numerous research projects on deafness, quality of life, mental health, deaf adults and pupils.

ANA GARCÍA GARCÍA is a clinical psychologist and Spanish Sign Language interpreter. She was co-founder of the Spanish Society for Mental Health & Deafness, and council member of the European Society for Mental Health and Deafness (ESMHD) since 1995. Since 2001, she has been coordinator and clinical psychologist at the Mental Health Unit for the Deaf at the general hospital "Gregorio Marañón" in Madrid, Spain, and since 2010, co-chair of the Medical Issues Special Interest Group of the ESMHD. She has conducted numerous research projects and lectures on mental health and deafness.

KIKA HADJIKAKOU, PH.D, is qualified teacher of the deaf, CSL interpreter, and PhD holder in deaf education, currently working as a special needs coordinator at the Cyprus Ministry of Education and Culture. She is also employed as a visiting lecturer at the European University of Cyprus. She has published numerous papers and chapters in international journals and books on deaf education, Deaf culture, inclusion, families with deaf children, and so forth.

JOANNA KOBOSKO, PH.D., is a clinical pychologist, working at the Institute of Physiology and Pathology of Hearing, Warsaw, Poland since 1996. Her professional interests focus on hearing parents of deaf and hard of hearing children, deaf adolescents' identity development, and in recent years, on the psychological functioning of postlingually deaf adults using cochlear implants. Her scientific attainments include editorship of several collective works on deafness (most recently, *Deaf and Hard of Hearing Adolescents in Their Families and Environment*) and many scientific and popular science articles on the psychological functioning of deaf children and adolescents and their families. She is a lecturer in postgraduate studies for pedagogues, psychologists, and speech therapists, preparing them for working with the deaf and hard of hearing. Since 1999, she has represented Poland at the ESMHD congresses and special interest groups, and since 2008, has been a member of the ESMHD Council. Since 2012, she has been a general secretary of the journal *Nowa Audiofonologia*.

POORNA KUSHALNAGAR, PH.D., is a Deaf first-generation American of hearing immigrant Indian parents, and a research associate professor at the Rochester Institute of Technology. She is the Director of Deaf Health Communication and Quality of Life Center, where she continues to conduct health and quality of life research with deaf and hard of hearing people across the lifespan. Her work has been funded by government agencies including the National Institute of Health and Department of Education.

IRENE W. LEIGH, PH.D., is a Deaf psychologist, she received a bachelor's degree in Deaf education from Northwestern University, and two master's degrees (one in rehabilitation counseling and one in psychology) as well as a Ph.D. in clinical psychology, all from New York University. Currently she is professor emerita of psychology, having worked in the doctoral program in clinical psychology at Gallaudet University and chaired its Department of Psychology. Her research interests and extensive publications are related to the measurement of depression among deaf people, identity and multiculturalism, parenting, parent-child attachment, and cochlear implants. She is a fellow of the American Psychological Association and former associate editor of the *Journal of Deaf Studies and Deaf Education*.

GEORGINA MITRE FAJARDO has a master's degree in habilitation and rehabilitation of persons with disabilities from the University of Salamanca (Spain) and a degree in psychology from the Universidad Autonoma de San Luis Potosí (Mexico). She is an independent researcher in the field of autism and is currently studying for her "quality doctorate" at the University of Salamanca on "Advances in research and perspectives on disability." She has conducted research on deaf adolescents and sexuality, and eye contact and imitation skills in children with autism. She is currently working on funded research and multidisciplinary collaborative projects with international researchers. Her current research is on communication skills in prelinguistic children with autism.

JAVIER MUÑOZ BRAVO is a clinical psychologist. He holds a master's degree in health economics and health management and master's degree in administration and health services management. He is a Spanish Sign Language interpreter, and founder of the Spanish Society for Mental Health and Deafness. He was an executive member of the European Society for Mental Health and Deafness from 2004 till 2010. He has conducted numerous research projects on deafness, disability, general and mental health, and is currently editor of the *International Journal on Mental Health & Deafness*.

DONALD L. PATRICK, PH.D., is the director of the Seattle Quality of Life Group and professor of Health Services at the University of Washington School of Public Health.

ANNE SKALICKY, M.S., is a hearing professional who lived two and a half years in Guatemala, and currently lives in the Seattle area. She served as a research scientist on the National Institute of Health R01 Quality of Life grant for deaf and hard of hearing youth from 2009 to 2010.

INES (CJ.) SLEEBOOM-VAN RAAIJ, M.D., is a consultant psychiatrist of the Royal Kentalis Group in the Netherlands since April 2009, of the mental health service for the deaf, Trajectum Hoeve Boschoord (forensic mental health and deafness), and Odion, Philadelphia, and Zaam (supraregional services for supported living). In 1984 she was the first psychiatrist in the Netherlands interested in mental health and deafness. She was the founder and medical director from 1990 until 2009 of VIA National Centre for Mental Health and Auditive Disorders, and consultant psychiatrist of the Riethorst Mental Health Service for the Deaf from 2009 until 2015. She is trained in client-centered psychotherapy (Rogers), cognitive behavioral psychotherapy, family therapy, directive therapy, forensic assessment, psychopharmacology, and research issues. She has been president of the European Society Mental Health and Deafness (ESMHD) since 2007, founder and coordinator of the Medical Issues Special Interest group and an executive member of the ESMHD since 2003. She was co-president of the seventh ESMHD Congress in Haarlem, the Netherlands and the 6th World Congress in 2014 in Belfast, Northern Ireland. She has written multiple publications about various aspects of mental health and deafness, tinnitus, and hyperacusis.

KAREN A. TINSLEY, M.A., CI, NIC, NCC, LPC, is a Hard of Hearing national certified counselor and RID certified interpreter, who received a bachelor's degree in psychology from Northeastern University, and a master's degree in counseling (mental health) from Gallaudet University. Her clinical experiences include case management and counseling in both inpatient and outpatient deaf programs, as well as several residential schools for the deaf. She also worked as an educational interpreter for seven years and has published articles in the RID newsletter including, "Working with Special Needs Students," a linguistic analysis of a Deaf student with autism. Her current practice interests are related to fostering culturally sensitive equine-assisted counseling and furthering the field through her study of The Art Of Riding®, and how the fields of psychology, neuroscience, and energy-work contribute to its evolution as an effective treatment option.

TIEJO VAN GENT, MD, PH.D., is a consultant child and adolescent psychiatrist specialized in mental health issues of deaf and hard of hearing children, and children with speech and language disorders. He co-founded one of the first specialized in- and outpatient mental health services for deaf and hard of hearing children and young people worldwide. His research concerns the prevalence of mental health problems in deaf and hard of hearing children and adolescents, and associations between intrapersonal factors such as self-concept and ego development, putative chronic stressors and emotional and behavioral health disorders. Since 2008 he has worked as a consultant at Royal Dutch Kentalis which provides diagnostics, care and educational services to deaf and hard of hearing individuals, nationwide.

Index

on national health budgets, 41–42
quality of life research instrument from,
114
on right to health, 3

Young, A., 199
youth quality of life (YQoL), 131–32,
134–37, 135*t*, 138. *See also* Deaf

children and adolescents; hearing
children and adolescents
Youth Self-Report (YSR), 197

Zalewska, Marina, 198, 200
Zea, M. C., 90
zuclopenthixol, 24